MCQs in
Otolaryngology
and
Head and Neck Surgery

To Lorraine and Lucy

MCQs in Otolaryngology and Head and Neck Surgery

Jack M. Lancer MB ChB(Sheffield), LRCP, MRCS, FRCS(Eng), DLO
Consultant in Otolaryngology, Rotherham Health Authority; Honorary Clinical
Lecturer, University of Sheffield

and

Andrew S. Jones MB BCh(Wales), MD, FRCS(Ed)
Senior Lecturer in Otorhinolargngology, University of Liverpool; Honorary
Consultant in Otorhinolargngology, Walton Hospital, Liverpool

Butterworths
London Boston Singapore Sydney Toronto Wellington

First published, 1988

© **Butterworth & Co. (Publishers) Ltd, 1988**

British Library Cataloguing in Publication Data

Lancer, Jack M. (Jack Michael)
  MCQs in otolaryngology and head and
  neck surgery
  1. Otolaryngology – Questions & Answers.
  2. Man. Head & neck. Surgery
  I. Title II. Jones, Andrew S.
  616.2'2'0074

ISBN 0-407-00761-X

Library of Congress Cataloging in Publication Data

Lancer, Jack M.
  MCQs in otolaryngology and head and neck surgery.
  1. Otolaryngology – Examinations, questions, etc.
  2. Head – Surgery – Examinations, questions, etc.
  3. Neck – Surgery – Examinations, questions, etc.
  I. Jones, Andrew S. II. Title. [DNLM: 1. Head
  – surgery – examination questions. 2. Neck – surgery
  – examination questions. 3. Otorhinolaryngologic
  Diseases – examination questions. WV 18 L247m]

RF57.L36 1988   617'.51'0076   88-16704
ISBN 0-407-00761-X

Typeset and Printed by The Alden Press, Oxford, London and Northampton

FOREWORD

The practice of medicine is a continuing process of learning. We are taught formally by lectures or in clinics, at the bedside or in the laboratory; or we teach ourselves by reading or watching teaching programmes using slides or video tapes.

To have been taught is one thing, to have learned is another. Formal examinations are necessary in medicine to confirm that the student's knowledge has reached a satisfactory and safe level. The discipline of honest self-examination is equally desirable, though less easily arranged.

The present volume offers an opportunity to otolaryngology students of all ages to test their present store of knowledge comprehensively.

The student who uses this book without self-deception may derive satisfaction or alarm from his or her performance. In either case, the endeavour should prove to be a most untrivial pursuit!

J.T. Buffin
Head of Otolaryngology Department
Royal Hallamshire Hospital and The Children's Hospital
Sheffield

PREFACE

In this book, our aim has been to base multiple choice questions on those aspects of otorhinolaryngology which have most relevance to clinical practice. It was the absence of such a book that prompted us to write this volume.

At present, multiple choice questions do not figure in Part 2 of the Fellowship examinations of the Royal College of Surgeons (FRCS). They do, however, play a role in the first part. For this reason, a large proportion of the contents of the book is devoted to such basic and applied anatomy as is relevant to the otolaryngologist. Multiple choice questions are a useful method of self-assessment and, indeed, it is to this end that the book is designed.

The book is not divided into separate sections, nor is each question related to the previous or following question. Thus it is hoped that the reader will always be on his or her toes, wondering what the subject of the next question will be rather than settling down to a rhinology section, for example.

We have endeavoured to cover all relevant aspects of otolaryngological practice but we apologize for any omissions or ambiguities. The subjects covered include otology, audiology, rhinology (including allergy), laryngology (including head and neck cancer surgery), relevant pharmacology, physiology, anatomy, microbiology and pathology, and a few other miscellaneous – and possibly humorous – questions for which no specific category is appropriate.

Each question consists of a common stem giving rise to five branches. The stem and a single branch together constitute an independent statement, to be judged as 'true' or 'false' by the reader. Thus five independent decisions are required in order to answer each question. This system has the advantage over other forms of multiple choice questions of being simple, yet concise.

When attempting each question the reader should award himself or herself one mark for each correct answer, deduct one mark for each incorrect answer, and take no score if the question is not answered. Three or more marks per question out of the maximum of five represents a 'pass'.

We hope that you will derive some pleasure – and at least a little knowledge – from attempting to answer the questions and we wish you all the best of luck!

J.M.L
A.S.J
February 1988

1 **The flexible fibreoptic rhinolaryngoscope:**
  A   Use of this instrument enables a thorough assessment of the upper respiratory tract to be carried out during general anaesthesia
  B   Can pass along the eustachian tube
  C   Is recommended for obtaining laryngeal biopsies
  D   Visualization to the carina is possible in the majority of patients
  E   Has a 180° field of view

2 **Vocal cord nodules (singers' nodules):**
  A   May become malignant
  B   Are always bilateral
  C   Respond favourably to speech therapy in most patients
  D   Are related to alcohol consumption
  E   Should be removed by microsurgical techniques soon after their diagnosis

3 **The frontal sinus:**
  A   Symmetry is usual on left and right
  B   Receives its nerve supply via the maxillary nerve
  C   Is the second commonest sinus for the development of a benign osteoma
  D   Drains via its duct into the superior meatus
  E   May be congenitally absent

4 **Causes of nasal obstruction include:**
  A   Aspirin ingestion
  B   Atrophic rhinitis
  C   Menthol inhalation
  D   Topical anaesthesia with lignocaine
  E   Xylometazoline spray

5 **The glossopharyngeal nerve:**
  A   Is the nerve of the second branchial arch
  B   Is motor to the intrinsic lingual muscles
  C   Is motor to some extrinsic lingual muscles
  D   Supplies sensation to the middle ear mucous membrane
  E   Is deep to the tonsil fossa

2 Answers

1 A F Examination with this endoscope under local anaesthesia is an indispensible outpatient procedure. Function cannot easily be assessed under a general anaesthetic.
   B F The instrument in common usage has a tip diameter of 3.4 mm, and cannot therefore pass along the eustachian tube.
   C F In the standard model there is no biopsy channel present. Ideally, laryngeal biopsies should not take place in an outpatient setting.
   D T All areas from the nasal vestibule to the carina may be viewed.
   E F The field of view is 85°.

2 A F There is no known association.
   B F Although bilateral nodules are more usual, unilateral nodules do occur.
   C T Treatment for singers' nodules that includes speech therapy has a more favourable outcome. It should always be used as a primary therapy.
   D F There is no proven relationship.
   E F A trial with speech therapy should be undertaken initially. Surgery should only be undertaken if the nodules fail to respond. Speech therapy should be continued after surgery.

3 A F The frontal sinuses are usually asymmetrical.
   B F Sensation is supplied by the frontal branch of the ophthalmic division of the trigeminal nerve.
   C F Routine radiology of the frontal sinuses shows evidence of osteomas in at least 1% of patients. The frontal sinus is the commonest, followed by the ethmoidal, the maxillary and the sphenoidal sinuses.
   D F The frontonasal duct drains into the middle meatus.
   E T This finding is not uncommon, thus X-rays are essential prior to undertaking surgery for suspected frontal sinus disease.

4 A T Most prostaglandins are nasal decongestants. Aspirin inhibits prostaglandin synthesis thereby causing nasal obstruction.
   B T Although the nasal cavity is invariably voluminous in atrophic rhinitis, the sensation of nasal obstruction may be due to the destruction of peripheral nerve endings.
   C F Menthol causes a subjective improvement in nasal patency.
   D F Lignocaine causes a subjective improvement in nasal patency.
   E T Following an initial improvement in nasal patency there may be a rebound nasal congestion.

5 A F It is the nerve of the third branchial arch.
   B F
   C F The glossopharyngeal nerve is motor to only one muscle, the stylopharyngeus.
   D T And also to the carotid body, the oropharynx, with taste to the posterior third of the tongue, and carries secretomotor fibres to the parotid gland.
   E T It may be sectioned by a tonsillectomy approach for glossopharyngeal neuralgia.

6 **Recurrent laryngeal nerve paralysis:**
   A A cause is found in over 90% of cases
   B Is commoner on the left side
   C If the patient is hoarse and the paralysis is unilateral, teflon injection is advised at an early stage
   D May occur following influenza
   E Laryngectomy is a recognized treatment

7 **Indications for the Caldwell–Luc operation include:**
   A Recurrent 'allergic' nasal polyposis
   B Orbital 'blow out' fracture
   C Biopsy for suspected antral malignancy
   D Recurrent epistaxis
   E Recurrent attacks of chronic maxillary sinusitis

8 **The Alder–Hey tracheostomy tube:**
   A Has a fenestrated outer tube
   B Consists of five pieces
   C Is more commonly used in adults
   D Is cuffed
   E Is so-called because of the name of its designer

9 **'Dysphonia' is:**
   A The decreased ability to vocalize because of cerebral dysfunction
   B The decreased ability to vocalize because of an abnormality of the articulating mechanism
   C The decreased ability to vocalize because of a laryngeal disorder
   D Difficulty in swallowing
   E The decreased ability to vocalize because of prolonged vocal abuse, such as long telephone conversations

10 **Indications for tonsillectomy:**
   A Two severe attacks of acute tonsillitis in a year
   B Psoriasis
   C Carriers of *Staphylococcus aureus*
   D Recurrent acute otitis media
   E Sleep apnoea due to gross tonsillar hypertrophy

4 Answers

6   A F 50% are idiopathic.
    B T Because the left recurrent laryngeal nerve has a longer course running through the chest.
    C F There should be a delay of 6 months except when the palsy is due to a malignant growth since spontaneous recovery may occur.
    D T But may recover.
    E T For bilateral adductor paralysis, especially if aspiration is a problem.

7   A F The problem originates in the ethmoid sinuses.
    B T
    C F Such a biopsy should preferably be performed via an intranasal antrostomy so that tumour seeding is minimized.
    D T
    E T Other indications include the removal of foreign bodies (teeth), dental cysts involving the antrum, and antrochoanal polypi; as an approach to the pterygopalatine fossa to ligate the maxillary artery and perform Vidian neurectomy; and to approach the posterior ethmoidal air cells (Horgan's operation).

8   A T
    B T It consists of an outer tube, two inner tubes (one with a speaking valve), an introducer and a 'blocker'.
    C F It is primarily for use in children.
    D F
    E F it is so named after the hospital where it was designed.

9   A F This is dysphasia.
    B F This is dysarthria.
    C T Dysphonia is the special example of dysarthria, from faulty working of the vocal cords.
    D F This is dysphagia.
    E F

10 A F Conventional teaching states that there should be 4–5 attacks per year for at least 2 years.
    B T Possibly by an alteration in the immune response.
    C F It should be considered in carriers of the β-haemolytic streptococcus if it cannot be eradicated with antibiotics, especially in high-risk groups, such as operating theatre workers.
    D T If attacks of acute otitis media occur with attacks of tonsillitis, tonsillectomy may then be indicated.
    E T Other indications include neoplasms, rheumatic fever or acute glomerulonephritis associated with streptococcal tonsillitis, peritonsillar, parapharyngeal or retropharyngeal abscesses, and as an approach to the tonsil fossa to section the glossopharyngeal nerve or to remove the styloid process.

11 **Causes of a cartilaginous nasal septal perforation include:**
    A   Syphilis
    B   Cocaine sniffing
    C   Nose picking
    D   Wegener's granulomatosis
    E   Asbestos inhalation

12 **Otosclerosis:**
    A   Is autosomal recessive
    B   Is invariably unilateral
    C   Usually presents in the fifth decade
    D   May progress rapidly during pregnancy
    E   Is helped by treatment with sodium fluoride

13 **The lateral semicircular canal:**
    A   Shares a crus with the superior semicircular canal to open into the vestibule
    B   Shares a crus with the posterior semicircular canal to open into the vestibule
    C   Transmits via the superior vestibular nerve
    D   Is directly related to the first bend of the facial canal in the temporal bone (genu)
    E   Is an important landmark for the operation of saccus decompression

14 **Features of Horner's syndrome include:**
    A   Ipsilateral pupil dilatation
    B   Ipsilateral ptosis
    C   Ipsilateral facial sweating
    D   Ipsilateral facial flushing
    E   Exophthalmos

15 **The following structures are removed in the operation of radical neck dissection:**
    A   Sternomastoid
    B   Trapezius
    C   External carotid artery
    D   Internal jugular vein
    E   Sympathetic chain

16 **Sensory nerves of the ear include:**
    A   Mandibular nerve
    B   Glossopharyngeal nerve
    C   Lesser occipital nerve
    D   Cranial accessory nerve
    E   Maxillary nerve

6 Answers

11   A F Syphilis typically causes a bony septal perforation.
     B T Other causes include iatrogenic (postoperative) disorders, tumours,
     C T workers with cadmium, nickel, chromium or those in dusty environ-
     D T ments, and other chronic inflammatory disorders (TB, leprosy,
     E T sarcoid and fungal disorders).

12   A F It is an autosomal dominant disorder with incomplete penetrance.
     B F Otosclerosis is usually bilateral but it is unilateral in 11–15% of
         patients.
     C F It may present from 5 years to over 50 years but the initial complaint
         of hearing loss is most common in the third decade.
     D T Up to 50% may notice a progression of the hearing loss during
         pregnancy.
     E T In selected cases sodium fluoride may be of value, causing
         maturation of the diseased bone and arresting the development or
         progression of associated sensorineural deafness.

13   A F The crus commune is shared by the superior and the posterior
     B F semicircular canals.
     C T This nerve also transmits from the superior semicircular canal and
         the utricle.
     D F It is at the second bend where the facial nerve is situated, between
         the lateral semicircular canal and the oval window.
     E T So are the posterior semicircular canal and the sigmoid sinus.

14   A F There is pupil constriction due to unchecked parasympathetic
         activity since Horner's syndrome results from interruption of the
         cervical sympathetic chain.
     B T This is partial since the levator palpebrae superioris muscle also
         receives a motor supply from the oculomotor nerve.
     C F Sweat glands are under sympathetic control.
     D T There is vasodilatation.
     E F There may be enophthalmos.

15   A T Other structures removed or divided include omohyoid, the access-
     B F ory nerve, the cervical lymph nodes and the submandibular gland.
     C F
     D T
     E F

16   A T Via the auricular branch of the auriculotemporal nerve.
     B T This supplies the mucous membrane of the middle ear (Jacobson's
         nerve).
     C T Others include the great auricular nerve and the auricular branch of
         the vagus (Arnold's nerve).
     D F
     E F

17 **The following associations occur:**
A Squamous carcinoma of the antro-ethmoid region and woodworkers
B Postcricoid carcinoma and vitamin B_{12} deficiency anaemia
C Sarcoidosis and nasal septal saddle deformity
D Squamous cell carcinoma of the nasopharynx and inhabitants of Canton, China
E Lyme disease and Lucerne, Switzerland

18 **Saliva:**
A The total volume per day is 0.5–1.0 litres
B Secretion is decreased by opiate administration
C Flow from the parotid gland is regulated from the inferior salivatory nucleus in the medulla
D Has only the functions of moistening the mouth and an antibacterial effect
E Has a mean pH of 7.5

19 **Typical findings in Menière's disease:**
A Sensorineural deafness affecting mainly the low tones in the early stages of the disease
B Loudness balance testing showing recruitment
C The presence of tone decay
D A tympanometry curve showing a negative middle ear pressure
E Speech audiometry reaching 100%

20 **Cortical mastoidectomy may be performed for the following:**
A As a preliminary for a translabyrinthine approach to the internal auditory canal
B Exposure of the tympanic part of the facial nerve
C A facial paralysis associated with acute otitis media
D Bell's palsy
E Serous otitis media

21 **Branches of the external carotid artery include:**
A Inferior thyroid
B Transverse cervical
C Facial
D Ophthalmic
E Ascending pharyngeal

8 Answers

17   A F Adenocarcinoma of this area affects woodworkers and cobblers.

      B T Plummer–Vinson syndrome is associated with postcricoid carcinoma and, in this syndrome, 60% have a microcytic anaemia and 10% have a low serum vitamin B_{12}.

      C T As with other chronic granulomatous disorders, the nasal septum may be affected leading to a dorsal collapse.

      D T In Canton, South China, this is the most common cancer in men, constituting 57% of all cancers in that sex.

      E T Lyme disease is due to a spirochaete and, although originating in the USA, there is a high incidence in Lucerne. It may present to the otolaryngologist as a facial palsy.

18   A T

      B F Opiates induce nausea and this is almost always accompanied by an increase in salivation.

      C T And the superior salivatory nucleus regulates the flow from the submandibular and sublingual glands.

      D F Other functions include a cleansing and digestive action, lubrication in swallowing and speech, buffering, diluent and solvent action, and a role in the thirst mechanism.

      E F The mean pH is 6.7 (range 5.6–7.6) but it is sensitive to changes in salivary flow rate.

19   A T

      B T It may also show over-recruitment.

      C F As Menière's disease is an end-organ disorder, there should be no auditory adaptation when a sound of 4000 Hz is used for 60 s, 20 dB above the auditory threshold.

      D F The middle ear is not affected by the disorder.

      E F There is decreased speech discrimination but this is not as severe as in neural lesions.

20   A T Otherwise access to the internal auditory meatus would not be possible.

      B F Access would be too limited and a tympanotomy or a 'canal wall down' procedure would be required.

      C F Surgery is indicated if acute mastoiditis supervenes.

      D F Treatment is usually conservative but if surgery was to be performed, then a total nerve decompression from the internal auditory meatus to the styloid process should be considered.

      E T In persistent cases.

21   A F Other branches include the superior thyroid, lingual, occipital,

      B F posterior auricular, superficial temporal and maxillary arteries.

      C T

      D F

      E T

22 **Fractures of the petrous temporal bone:**
    A   Are longitudinal in 80% of cases
    B   A facial paralysis is commoner if the fracture is transverse
    C   Blood clot in the external ear canal should be removed and the tympanic membrane inspected
    D   Cerebrospinal fluid leaks invariably need surgical closure
    E   Bleeding from the external auditory meatus usually occurs in longitudinal fractures

23 **The facial nerve:**
    A   Is motor to the tensor tympani muscle
    B   In the internal auditory canal lies inferior to the cochlear nerve
    C   Is the nerve in the internal auditory meatus to be most frequently affected by a neuroma
    D   Lies over the ampulla of the posterior semicircular canal
    E   Its first branch is the greater superficial petrosal nerve

24 **Gradenigo's syndrome:**
    A   Occurs because of petrosal inflammation or purulent accumulation
    B   Includes an abducent nerve paralysis
    C   Includes pain
    D   Includes facial paralysis
    E   Includes tinnitus

25 **Tuberculosis of the larynx:**
    A   Usually occurs secondarily to tuberculous lesions elsewhere in the body
    B   May lead to irreversible laryngeal scarring
    C   Is no longer seen in the UK
    D   Laryngoscopy may show a unilateral red vocal cord
    E   Treatment is surgical

26 **In the internal auditory meatus:**
    A   The cochlear nerve is medial to the inferior vestibular nerve
    B   The facial nerve is lateral to the superior vestibular nerve
    C   The inferior vestibular nerve is inferior to the cochlear nerve
    D   The superior vestibular nerve is medial to the inferior vestibular nerve
    E   'Bill's Bar' separates the facial and superior vestibular nerve from the cochlear and inferior vestibular nerve

22   A T And transverse in 20% of cases.
     B T As the fracture usually goes through the otic capsule.
     C F Blood clot acts as a good dressing and should be left alone in the majority of cases.
     D F Most CSF leaks close spontaneously within 7–10 days.
     E T Because the skin of the external ear canal and the tympanic membrane are frequently torn. In transverse fractures there is usually a haemotympanum but no bleeding from the ear.

23   A F This muscle is supplied by a branch of the mandibular nerve.
     B F It is superior.
     C F This honour goes to the superior vestibular nerve.
     D T It can be damaged at this site while skeletonizing the posterior semicircular canal.
     E T This is given off at the genu.

24   A T
     B T The nerve is compressed by oedema where it passes through Dorello's canal beneath the petrosphenoid ligament (of Grüber) at the tip of the petrous apex.
     C T The site of the pain depends on whether there is an anterior or a posterior petrositis, and is due to pressure forward against the dural envelope of the Gasserian ganglion since it lies just anterior to the petrous tip.
     D F Facial paralysis and tinnitus are not a part of the syndrome. The triad
     E F is completed by a discharging ear.

25   A T It is usually secondary to pulmonary tuberculosis.
     B T This finding may be encountered many years after the disease has been cured.
     C F Tuberculosis should always be considered in the differential diagnosis of otolaryngological disorders.
     D T The differential diagnosis of a unilateral red vocal cord should also include a malignant growth and syphilis.
     E F After the diagnosis is confirmed following a biopsy, treatment is medical with a prolonged course of appropriate antibiotics.

26   A T In the internal auditory meatus the facial nerve is superior and
     B F medial, the cochlear nerve is inferior and medial, the superior
     C F vestibular nerve is superior and lateral, and the inferior vestibular
     D F nerve is inferior and lateral.
     E F The horizontal (falciform) crest does this. 'Bill's Bar', named after William House of Los Angeles, is a vertical bar of bone separating the facial nerve from the superior vestibular nerve.

27   **A deviated nasal septum:**
  A   Usually causes symptoms
  B   May predispose to ipsilateral chronic otitis media
  C   Should be corrected by a submucosal resection of the nasal septum
  D   The commonest cause is trauma
  E   The vomerine bone invariably contributes to the deviation

28   **Indications for tracheostomy:**
  A   Angioneurotic oedema of the larynx
  B   A right vocal cord paralysis
  C   Respiratory insufficiency caused by muscular disease
  D   Electively, prior to a radical neck dissection
  E   Tetanus

29   **The following nerves are sensory to the teeth:**
  A   Mental
  B   Anterior superior alveolar
  C   Anterior palatine
  D   Lingual
  E   Lesser superficial petrosal

30   **Benign tumours of the larynx:**
  A   Constitute approximately 20% of all laryngeal tumours
  B   Papillomata are the commonest
  C   Papillomata are usually solitary before puberty
  D   Juvenile papillomata are associated with maternal condylomata acuminata
  E   The treatment of choice for juvenile papillomata is excision with the carbon dioxide laser

12   Answers

27   A   F In many people a deviated nasal septum is a chance finding and is asymptomatic. Very few people have a straight nasal septum.

B   T The classical teaching is that a deviated nasal septum may predispose to or aggravate chronic otitis media, possibly because of the decreased airflow through the affected side with a subsequent deleterious effect on eustachian tube function.

C   F Most deviated nasal septa are asymptomatic and therefore surgery is not required. However, if the deviation is thought to be the cause of symptoms it may be corrected by a submucosal resection of the nasal septum (SMR) or a septoplasty.

D   F Most are thought to be congenital and are affected by growth. Traumatic deviations form a small group.

E   T Although symptomatic deviations are chiefly due to a cartilaginous deformity. The more anterior the deformity, the greater the symptoms.

28   A   T In this instance, tracheostomy may be life-saving, especially if adrenaline and endotracheal intubation are unavailable.

B   F As long as the contralateral vocal cord is working normally there is usually an adequate airway.

C   T To enable intermittent positive pressure respiration, which will reduce the airflow resistance and the volume of the dead space.

D   F But may be required as an elective procedure prior to surgery on the larynx, pharynx, mandible and oral cavity.

E   T To allow for controlled respiration following planned drug-induced paralysis of the respiratory musculature.

29   A   T The nerve supply of the teeth of the upper jaw is by the alveolar
B   T branches of the maxillary nerve and that of the lower jaw is by the
C   F inferior alveolar branch of the mandibular division of the trigeminal
D   F nerve.
E   F

30   A   F True benign tumours of the larynx constitute less than 5% of all laryngeal tumours.

B   T Papillomata constitute 85% of benign laryngeal tumours.

C   F They are usually multiple before puberty – juvenile papillomatosis – and may regress around puberty. The adult type is usually solitary and does not undergo spontaneous regression.

D   T Mothers who are known to have genital warts at the time of delivery may be advised to undergo an elective caesarean section.

E   T But other treatments are still performed and these include removal under general anaesthesia via direct laryngoscopy (often under microscopic vision) and sometimes using suction diathermy.

31 **Following tonsillectomy:**
- A   Otalgia will always be due to referred pain from the tonsil fossa
- B   Secondary haemorrhage can occur at 48 h
- C   The treatment of secondary haemorrhage is usually conservative
- D   In a sleeping patient, the most reliable physical sign for detection of a reactionary haemorrhage is a fall in the blood pressure
- E   Temporomandibular joint dysfunction may occur

32 **Complications of tonsillitis include:**
- A   Tonsillar haemorrhage
- B   Parapharyngeal abscess
- C   Cor pulmonale
- D   Serous otitis media
- E   Renal failure

33 **Tumours of the thyroid gland:**
- A   Anaplastic carcinoma typically metastasises by haematogenous spread
- B   Papillary carcinoma typically metastasises by haematogenous spread
- C   Medullary carcinomas are associated with phaeochromocytomas
- D   A history of irradiation to the neck in fetal life or childhood may be a predisposing factor
- E   A malignant lymphoma is the most likely thyroid neoplasm to become calcified

34 **Ostia of the nasal sinuses:**
- A   The ostium of the posterior ethmoidal group is in the middle meatus
- B   The sphenoidal sinus ostium is in the superior meatus
- C   The accessory maxillary sinus ostium is in the superior meatus
- D   The maxillary sinus ostium is situated within the middle meatus
- E   The ostium of the anterior ethmoidal group is in the inferior meatus

35 **The rigid bronchoscope:**
- A   Usually allows detection of neoplasms of the upper lobe bronchi
- B   Can detect most small bronchial neoplasms
- C   Can be easily used by anyone with an interest in endoscopy of the bronchi
- D   Is the best instrument for the removal of a bronchial foreign body
- E   Bronchoscopy is easily performed under local anaesthesia

14   Answers

31   A F Acute otitis media may complicate tonsillectomy and all patients with postoperative otalgia need otoscopic examination.
      B T But it would be more usual between 7–10 days.
      C T It is usually due to infection and is treated by antibiotics, intravenous infusions and with blood if necessary. In severe cases surgery may be required.
      D F This sign occurs relatively late. A rising pulse and frequent swallowing are much more reliable.
      E T From hyperextension of the mandible by the mouth gag, especially in adults.

32   A T The mucous membrane overlying the tonsil may become so inflamed that spontaneous rupture of overlying vessels may occur.
      B T And also intratonsillar, peritonsillar and retropharyngeal abscesses.
      C T With gross tonsillar hypertrophy this complication may occur and will be exacerbated by repeated inflammatory episodes, perhaps necessitating a tracheostomy. There is usually an associated adenoidal hypertrophy, especially in children.
      D F However, this may occur following adenoidal swelling or inflammation, which usually occurs concurrently with tonsillitis.
      E T Acute glomerulonephritis may occur due to the production of anti-streptococcal antibodies, which react adversely with the glomerular basement membrane.

33   A F It infiltrates the surrounding tissues causing pain and hoarseness and may compress the trachea giving stridor.
      B F Papillary carcinomas spread via the lymphatic stystem. Haematogenous spread is more characteristic of follicular carcinomas.
      C T The 'multiple endocrine adenomatosis 2' syndrome describes a pattern of endocrine malignancy, which also includes neuromas of the tongue, eyelids and lips, and parathyroid lesions.
      D T Ionizing radiation is carcinogenic in the developing thyroid gland.
      E F Medullary carcinomas tend to show calcification. They are derived from the C (calcitonin) cells.

34   A F Via their ostia, the sphenoidal sinus drains into the sphenoethmoidal
      B F recess, the posterior ethmoidal sinuses drain into the superior
      C F meatus, and the maxillary, frontal, anterior and middle ethmoidal
      D T sinuses drain into the middle meatus.
      E F

35   A F Even with a telescope, the detection range is limited to the hilar type of neoplasms or those located in the lobar, segmental and subsegmental bronchi of the middle and lower lobes.
      B F A majority of early small cancerous lesions are located in the branch bronchi of the upper lobes.
      C F Examination with this instrument requires much experience.
      D T Due to its large lumen.
      E F This is the case only in extremely skilled hands. It is more usual to perform such an examination under a general anaesthetic.

36   **The nasolacrimal duct:**
    A   Drains into the middle meatus
    B   The mouth of the duct is usually single
    C   The ostium is always round
    D   Usually opens 30–40 mm from the nostril
    E   The size of its orifice in the nose is usually less than 2 mm
        diameter

37   **The deltopectoral flap:**
    A   The upper margin is at the level of the clavicle
    B   The skin of the area from which the flap is obtained receives all
        its blood supply from the internal mammary artery
    C   The flap should always be 'delayed'
    D   Has numerous applications
    E   Should not be used if the patient has received prior radiotherapy
        for a head or neck neoplasm

38   **Central connections of the cochlear nerve include:**
    A   The superior olivary nucleus
    B   The medial geniculate body
    C   The lateral geniculate body
    D   The inferior colliculus
    E   The superior colliculus

39   **The constrictor muscles of the pharynx:**
    A   All have a motor nerve supply from the pharyngeal plexus
    B   Form a longitudinal layer of muscles around the pharynx
    C   The glossopharyngeal nerve enters the pharynx between the
        superior and the middle constrictor
    D   The upper border of the superior constrictor is free
    E   The middle constrictor arises from the greater and lesser cornua
        of the hyoid bone

40   **Lateral sinus thrombophlebitis complicated by acute otitis media:**
    A   The most constant symptom is fever
    B   Between bouts of fever the patient is alert and feels well
    C   Progressive anaemia may occur
    D   Signs of raised intracranial pressure may occur
    E   Is its commonest cause today

41   **Important landmarks for the operation of posterior tympanotomy:**
    A   Pyramid
    B   Posterior semicircular canal
    C   Chorda tympani
    D   Tympanic section of the facial nerve
    E   Descending (mastoid) section of the facial nerve

36   A F It opens into the inferior meatus.
      B T But may rarely be double, triple or quadruple.
      C F It may also be oval or slit-like.
      D T Rarely it will open further backward or forward.
      E F It is variable, ranging from a mere groove to a maximum of 10 mm.

37   A T The lower margin runs almost parallel as it proceeds from about the
            fifth costochondral junction to the apex of the anterior axillary fold.
      B F It also receives a blood supply from the acromiothoracic artery and,
            if the flap is a long one, from branches of the suprascapular and
            circumflex humeral arteries.
      C F Under ordinary circumstances 'delays' are seldom needed but there
            are exceptions when the patient is old and infirm, has diabetes mellitus
            or atherosclerosis; or, if an extra large flap is needed or when recon-
            struction is secondary or elective and a little time lost in the interest
            of added safety is of no great concern.
      D T It can attain a wide range of locations in the head and neck with a
            single move without recourse to intermediary movements of its
            pedicle.
      E F Usually the fields for such irradiation fall well above the donor area,
            leaving the flap unaffected. If low neck fields have been used, however,
            the radiation effect on its feeding vessels can be unpredictable.

38   A T Others include the cochlear nucleus, the lateral lemniscus and the
      B T auditory cortex.
      C F
      D T
      E F

39   A F The cricopharyngeal part of the inferior constrictor is supplied by the
            recurrent laryngeal nerve.
      B F They form a circular layer. The longitudinal layer includes stylo-
            pharyngeus, palatopharyngeus and salpingopharyngeus.
      C T
      D T It forms the lower boundary of the sinus of Morgagni, its upper
            border being the base of the skull.
      E T It also arises from the stylohyoid ligament.

40   A T There is usually a swinging pyrexia.
      B T Out of proportion to the seriousness of the illness.
      C T It is especially rapid and pronounced in haemolytic streptococcal
            infections.
      D T More commonly when the larger lateral sinus is thrombosed.
      E F The majority of cases today occur in chronic otorrhoea with
            cholesteatoma, and super-added acute infection.

41   A F The 'antrum threshold angle' needs to be removed. It is formed
      B F above by the fossa incudis, medially by the descending portion of
      C T the facial nerve and laterally by the chorda tympani.
      D F
      E T

42 **Ototoxicity:**
- A   The risk is increased by impaired renal function
- B   Gentamicin is primarily cochleotoxic
- C   The onset of deafness may be delayed following discontinuation of the drug
- D   Only occurs following parenteral drug administration
- E   Ototoxic deafness can be treated

43 **Acoustic neuromas:**
- A   Are usually unilateral
- B   Are the commonest tumours occurring in the cerebellopontine angle
- C   May present as sudden deafness
- D   Are treated with radiation
- E   Hearing may be preserved during tumour excision by the translabyrinthine route

44 **The pectoralis major myocutaneous flap:**
- A   Derives its axial blood supply from the thoracico-acromial artery
- B   Can be raised with an attached segment of rib to provide a vascularized bone graft
- C   A split skin graft is usually required for the donor site
- D   Can be used in a patient who has previously had a deltopectoral flap elevated from the same side of the chest
- E   Is very versatile

45 **Acoustic neuromas:**
- A   Histological examination demonstrates fusiform cells arranged in whorls
- B   Tympanometry is usually normal
- C   Most symptomatic tumours occur in old age
- D   Vestibular testing will usually detect an absent response on the involved side
- E   80% arise from the superior vestibular nerve

46 **The pterygopalatine ganglion:**
- A   Its parasympathetic root is from the lesser (superficial) petrosal nerve
- B   Branches of the maxillary nerve relay in the ganglion
- C   The sympathetic root enters the ganglion in the nerve of the pterygoid canal
- D   Supplies secretomotor activity to the mucous glands of the palate
- E   One of its branches passes through the palatovaginal canal

42 A T As most ototoxic drugs are eliminated in the urine, thus higher plasma levels may develop.
    B F It is primarily vestibulotoxic.
    C T There may be a long latent period. Deafness may initially be noted after the drug has been discontinued and may even progress for weeks or months.
    D F It may also occur following oral or topical administration.
    E F There is no effective treatment, although there have been reports of spontaneous recovery of hearing.

43 A T However, when occurring in patients with Von Recklinghausen's disease, they are often bilateral.
    B T They form over 80%. Others include meningiomas, cholesteatomas and rare tumours.
    C T In 20% of cases.
    D F Acoustic neuromas are histologically benign well-differentiated tumours and so radiation therapy and chemotherapy are not used. Surgical removal is usually recommended.
    E F But it may be by the middle fossa or retrosigmoid/retromastoid routes.

44 A T
    B T And may be used to replace a segment of mandible.
    C F Unless an extraordinarily large flap is elevated, primary closure of the donor site is usually accomplished.
    D T Because the axial blood supply deep to the muscle is not interrupted by the deltopectoral flap.
    E T It can reach most areas in the head and neck. It has sufficient bulk to fill cavities, to augment contour and to provide structured support.

45 A F This is the appearance of a meningioma. Acoustic neuromas show both densely and loosely cellular compact areas.
    B T But the stapedius reflex may have an altered threshold, may be absent or may decay.
    C F Most occur in middle age.
    D F It is usually reduced but seldom absent.
    E T 20% arise from the inferior vestibular nerve.

46 A F It is from the greater (superficial) petrosal nerve.
    B F The only cell bodies in the ganglion are parasympathetic.
    C T With the parasympathetic root.
    D T And also to the mucous glands of the nose, nasopharynx and sinuses, and the lacrimal gland.
    E T The pharyngeal nerve supplies the mucous membrane of the nasopharynx.

47 **Pleomorphic adenomas of the parotid gland:**
   A   Are characteristically painless, slow-growing and mobile
   B   A facial nerve weakness may be present in up to 25% of cases
   C   The majority of tumours occur in the tail of the parotid
   D   Occur more commonly than of the submandibular gland
   E   Are well encapsulated

48 **The auditory ossicles:**
   A   The stapes footplate is reniform
   B   The short process of the incus projects superiorly
   C   The tensor tympani tendon is inserted into the neck of the malleus
   D   The anterior crus of the stapes is shorter than the posterior crus
   E   The incudostapedial joint has a 'ball and socket' articulation

49 **Atrophic rhinitis:**
   A   Is characterized by a voluminous nasal cavity
   B   There may be a bacterial aetiology
   C   Used to be seen quite commonly in patients who had undergone radical nasal surgery for obstruction
   D   Can be cured by surgical closure of one or both nostrils
   E   The nasal mucous membrane undergoes metaplastic change from stratified squamous to ciliated columnar epithelium

50 **Choanal atresia:**
   A   May be acquired
   B   Is always apparent soon after birth
   C   As soon as the diagnosis is made, an emergency tracheostomy is required
   D   Is associated with other congenital abnormalities
   E   Is always due to the presence of a bony plate

51 **The branchial apparatus:**
   A   The nerve of the third branchial arch is the facial
   B   The digastric muscle is derived solely from the muscle mass of the mandibular (first) arch
   C   The three auditory ossicles are derived from the first arch cartilage
   D   The cricothyroid muscle is derived from the fourth branchial arch
   E   The stem of the stapedial artery is a remainder of the first aortic arch

52 **A $T_2N_2M_1$ glottic neoplasm would imply that:**
   A   Metastases, only above the diaphragm, are present
   B   Fixed homolateral lymph nodes only are present
   C   Both vocal cords may be fully mobile
   D   There may be reduced mobility of the vocal cords
   E   One or both vocal cords may be fixed

47   A   T
     B   F   It almost never occurs, and its occurrence suggests malignancy.
     C   F   Most occur in the lateral lobe, primarily under the lobule of the ear.
     D   T   The parotid gland accounts for approximately 80% of pleomorphic adenomas.
     E   F   There is a pseudocapsule and tumour 'pseudopodia' piercing the capsule are visible on histological examination.

48   A   T
     B   F   It projects posteriorly.
     C   F   It inserts into the upper end of the medial surface of the manubrium (handle) of the malleus.
     D   T
     E   T   And the malleoincudal joint has a 'saddle' articulation.

49   A   T   There is absorption of bone of the turbinates and lateral nasal walls.
     B   T   The aetiology is unknown but it is thought to be bacterial, at least in part.
     C   T   Recent work suggests that atrophic rhinitis no longer occurs following trimming of the inferior turbinates.
     D   T   The nostrils may be closed for several years and there is usually no recurrence when they are reopened (Young's operation).
     E   F   The converse is true.

50   A   T   Due to trauma, infection or radiotherapy.
     B   F   Only in bilateral cases.
     C   F   In bilateral cases the insertion of an oropharyngeal airway, pending definitive surgery, is all that is required.
     D   T   There is an increased incidence.
     E   F   The defect may also be membranous.

51   A   F   It is the glossopharyngeal.
     B   F   Only the anterior belly. The posterior belly is derived from the second branchial arch.
     C   F   The malleus and incus are. The stapes is derived from the cartilaginous element of the second branchial arch.
     D   T
     E   F   It is all that remains of the second aortic arch. The first aortic arch disappears completely.

52   A   F   A $T_2N_2M_1$ glottic neoplasm would imply that the tumour has
     B   F   extended from the glottis to the supraglottis or the subglottis, with
     C   T   normal or reduced vocal cord movement.
     D   T   Contralateral or bilateral regional lymph nodes are involved, which
     E   F   may or may not be fixed, and distant metastases are present.

53   **A saddle nose deformity:**
A   May occur following a septal haematoma
B   May occur following dislocation of the osseocartilaginous junction in the dorsal strut during septorhinoplasty
C   The best material for correction is silastic
D   It is essential for a bone graft to develop a blood supply
E   If occurring during septorhinoplasty it is usually due to the removal of too much of the deviated nasal septum

54   **The skull-base:**
A   The stylomastoid foramen transmits the facial nerve only
B   Foramen ovale transmits the middle meningeal artery
C   No structure passes completely through the foramen lacerum
D   Foramen magnum transmits the spinal roots of the accessory nerve
E   The lateral pterygoid plate gives origin to the pharyngobasilar fascia

55   **Beclomethasone dipropionate nasal spray:**
A   Delivers 50 mg in each metered dose
B   Its main use is in the prophylaxis and treatment of allergic rhinitis
C   Will ease the symptoms of nasal polyposis
D   May cause nasal irritation because the solvent used is polyethylene glycol
E   Should only be used with caution in subjects already on the pulmonary formulation of beclomethasone

56   **Nystagmus:**
A   Nystagmus without optic fixation is spontaneous nystagmus
B   Optic fixation abolishes central spontaneous nystagmus
C   For benign positional vertigo using Hallpike's positional test, nystagmus beats towards the downmost ear for a positive result, and,
D   The appearance of the nystagmus is not immediate
E   A warm water caloric test will induce nystagmus to the opposite ear

57   **Causes of a fluctuating hearing loss include:**
A   Serous otitis media
B   Otosclerosis
C   Acoustic neuroma
D   Multiple sclerosis
E   Otomandibular syndrome

53 A   T If there is subsequent infection there will invariably be chondral necrosis with subsequent collapse.

    B   T As well as traumatic and postoperative causes (e.g. a too radical SMR), saddling may occur as a congenital defect.

    C   F It is autogenous bone or cartilage. Silastic may erode through the nasal bridge skin.

    D   T In order to remain viable and prevent resection.

    E   F It is due to over-reduction of the nasal hump.

54 A   F It also transmits the stylomastoid branch of the posterior auricular artery.

    B   F It transmits the mandibular nerve and the accessory meningeal artery. The middle meningeal artery passes through the foramen spinosum.

    C   T However, the anterior orifice of the carotid canal opens on its posterior wall and the internal carotid artery then ascends through the upper end of the foramen.

    D   T These roots enter the skull via the foramen magnum and leave it with the cranial root via the jugular foramen.

    E   F It is the medial pterygoid plate.

55 A   F It is $50\,\mu g$.

    B   T It is also of value in non-allergic vasomotor rhinitis and nasal

    C   T polyposis. Small nasal polyps may regress and larger polyps may be controlled.

    D   F The nasal spray comes in two formulations. One contains freons, which may be irritant. The other is an aqueous preparation.

    E   F Systemic absorption from topical nasal and pulmonary applications, even with prolonged courses, is minimal and systemic effects are practically non-existent.

56 A   T

    B   F It is usually enhanced.

    C   T The nystagmus lasts for about 40 s and is also fatiguable. There is a

    D   T 5–10 s latent period prior to the onset of the nystagmus.

    E   F Remember 'COWS' – Cold Opposite, Warm Same.

57 A   T This is a frequently encountered cause of fluctuating conductive hearing loss. Cerumen obstruction of the ear canal is also common.

    B   F The hearing loss is slow and progressive with occasional episodes of rapid deterioration, as occurs during pregnancy.

    C   T A slowly progressive hearing loss is more usual and up to 20% may present with a sudden deafness. Fluctuating deafness can occur with small tumours.

    D   T The nature of the hearing loss does not follow a consistent pattern.

    E   T This syndrome also includes pain in and around the ear, fullness in the ear, tinnitus and a sensation of unsteadiness.

58 **Radiological features of acoustic neuromas:**
A   On tomography, the crista falciformis runs closer to the inferior wall of the internal auditory meatus than the superior wall
B   A CT scan without enhancement is adequate for visualization of most tumours
C   Magnetic Resonance Imaging (MRI) is useful in assessing tumour size
D   Air CT meatography is useful in demonstrating larger tumours
E   Air CT meatography may demonstrate the position of the anterior inferior cerebellar artery ('AICA')

59 **The following are useful investigations for allergic rhinitis:**
A   Eosinophil count in peripheral blood
B   Erythrocyte sedimentation rate (ESR)
C   Patch test
D   Culture of nasal secretions
E   PRIST (paper radioimmunosorbent test)

60 **Surgical approaches to the internal auditory meatus:**
A   The middle fossa approach should be used for extracanalicular tumours
B   The translabyrinthine approach can allow for hearing preservation
C   The translabyrinthine approach should be used for the removal of large intracanalicular tumours
D   The transotic approach affords excellent exposure of almost the entire internal auditory meatus
E   The retrolabyrinthine approach affords an excellent exposure of the last six cranial nerves

61 **Hypopharyngeal diverticula:**
A   Arise from a dehiscence between the middle and the inferior constrictor muscles
B   The diagnosis is usually confirmed by a barium swallow
C   Oesophagoscopy should be performed immediately prior to excision
D   A cricopharyngeal myotomy should be performed as a part of the procedure of external excision
E   Are associated with a hypochromic anaemia

62 **Indications for adenoidectomy:**
A   Cleft palate
B   Asymptomatic adenoidal enlargement
C   Sleep apnoea
D   Delayed speech development
E   Recurrent peritonsillar abscess

58   A T The crista falciformis normally lies at or above the midpoint of the vertical diameter of the canal.
      B F Most acoustic neuromas show some degree of contrast enhancement and will usually be present on the scan.
      C T MRI allows for a very accurate assessment of tumour shape, size and position.
      D F It is useful to outline smaller tumours in the cerebellopontine angle or confined to the meatus.
      E T And this is of surgical significance since the 'AICA' is intrameatal in 40% of patients.

59   A F Blood eosinophil count is only elevated in those patients also suffering from asthma.
      B F This is seldom elevated in uncomplicated allergic rhinitis.
      C F The scratch, prick and intracutaneous tests are useful.
      D T Along with sinus X-rays, this will help to eliminate sepsis as a cause of rhinitis.
      E T This measures total IgE and along with RAST (radioallergosorbent test), which measures allergen-specific IgE, are very useful.

60   A F It should be used for small intracanalicular tumours in the presence of serviceable hearing on the affected side.
      B F The labyrinth will be destroyed.
      C F Access for complete removal of large tumours in awkward when using the translabyrintrine approach solely.
      D T One is not restricted to the visualization of the posterolateral aspect of the internal auditory meatus by the transotic approach (an extended combined translabyrinthine and transcochlear approach).
      E F There is usually an excellent exposure of the V–IX cranial nerves only.

61   A F They arise posteriorly through a relatively unsupported part of the posterior pharyngeal wall (Killian's dehiscence) between the thyropharyngeal and cricopharyngeal parts of the inferior constrictor.
      B T The lower end of the oesophagus should also be examined to exclude an associated hiatus hernia.
      C T So that the presence of the pouch is confirmed, food debris is washed out, the pouch may be packed, and malignancy excluded.
      D T This procedure is said to lessen the chance of recurrence.
      E F Although in sideropenic dysphagia this finding is present in approximately 60% of patients.

62   A F It is essential to preserve the adenoids in such cases, unless they are causing severe problems.
      B F The adenoids usually regress in size from about the age of 6 years.
      C T Cor pulmonale and right heart failure may eventually ensue.
      D F Adenoidectomy is not thought to be of value.
      E F This is an indication for tonsillectomy.

63 **Oro-antral fistulae:**
  A   Most occur following dental extractions
  B   Small fistulae usually heal spontaneously
  C   Sinus X-rays are only of limited value
  D   Surgical repair of a fistula should be accompanied by a sinus
       drainage procedure
  E   Surgical closure is usually accomplished by primary apposition

64 **The endolymphatic sac:**
  A   Surgery to the sac is invariably followed by sensorineural
       deafness
  B   Surgery on the sac is performed for disabling vertigo from any
       cause which has not responded to medical therapy
  C   Successful surgery depends on the position of the sigmoid sinus
  D   Is usually situated medial to the sigmoid sinus and inferior to the
       posterior semicircular canal
  E   Donaldson's line is important in locating the sac

65 **In laryngomalacia (congenital laryngeal stridor):**
  A   Treatment is surgical
  B   Stridor is maximal during sleep
  C   The stridor is primarily due to a glottic disorder
  D   Laryngoscopy is indicated for diagnosis
  E   The supraglottis is usually normal

66 **The trachea:**
  A   Bifurcates into the left and right main bronchi usually at the
       level of the fifth thoracic vertebra
  B   Is encircled by cartilaginous rings
  C   The thyroid isthmus overlaps the fourth, fifth and sixth tracheal
       rings
  D   There are 8–10 cartilaginous rings
  E   The principal blood supply is from branches of the inferior
       thyroid artery

67 **Penicillin is usually the antibiotic of choice when treating infections
   caused by the following organisms:**
  A   *Actinomyces israelii*
  B   *Brucella abortus*
  C   *Mycoplasma pneumonii*
  D   *Bacillus anthracis*
  E   *Corynebacterium diphtheriae*

68 **The temporomandibular joint:**
  A   The articular surfaces are covered with hyaline cartilage
  B   An articular disc divides the joint into medial and lateral
       compartments
  C   The lateral pterygoid muscle helps to elevate the mandible
  D   Has a blood supply from the posterior auricular artery
  E   The coronoid process of the mandible articulates in the
       mandibular fossa

26 Answers

63 A T They may also occur following fractures, sinus surgery or may be
       associated with neoplasms or radiotherapy.
    B T If left undisturbed and infection does not supervene.
    C F They may demonstrate infection, retained roots or other foreign
       bodies, and neoplasms.
    D T The maxillary sinus is invariably infected.
    E F The fistula is usually too large for this and local mucosal flaps are
       required.

64 A F More destructive surgery is usually performed if saccus surgery is
       unsuccessful.
    B F Saccus surgery is usually performed only for Menière's disease.
    C T A very anteriorly situated sigmoid sinus may make access to the sac
       virtually impossible.
    D T
    E T This is an imaginary line in the plane of the lateral semicircular canal
       back towards the sigmoid sinus, and often marks the top end of the
       endolymphatic sac.

65 A F The stridor tends to disappear as the child grows.
    B T It may disappear when the child is active.
    C F It is produced by the supraglottis being sucked into the glottis during
       inspiration.
    D T To confirm the diagnosis and exclude other causes of stridor.
    E F There may be a normal-looking but floppy supraglottis. More
       commonly, however, the epiglottis is omega-shaped, the aryepiglottic
       folds are shortened, and the arytenoids are tall and slender.

66 A T It is the fourth thoracic vertebra in the cadaver.
    B F The first tracheal ring is the only one that is complete, the others
       being incomplete posteriorly.
    C F It lies over the second, third and fourth tracheal rings.
    D F The trachea has 16–20 cartilaginous rings.
    E T Its thoracic end is supplied from the bronchial arteries.

67 A T
    B F Tetracycline or co-trimoxazole is used.
    C F Tetracycline is effective.
    D T
    E T Penicillin would also be the antibiotic of choice in clostridial,
       treponemal, leptospiral and streptococcal infections.

68 A F They are covered with fibrocartilage.
    B F It divides the joint into upper and lower parts.
    C F This movement is produced by the temporalis, the medial pterygoid
       and the masseter muscles.
    D F It is from the superficial temporal and the maxillary arteries.
    E F It is the mandibular condyle which does this.

69 **Submandibular gland surgery may result in damage to the following nerves:**
A   Buccal branch of the facial nerve
B   Accessory nerve
C   Hypoglossal nerve
D   Lingual nerve
E   Recurrent laryngeal nerve

70 **The following otosurgical statements are correct:**
A   A homograft incus is the patient's own
B   A tympanic membrane will remain following a radical mastoidectomy
C   The posterior canal wall is left intact in a simple mastoidectomy
D   In a tympanoplasty there is always an attempt to restore or reconstruct the hearing mechanism
E   A combined approach tympanoplasty permits only the transmastoid removal of disease

71 **The atlas:**
A   Is the second cervical vertebrae
B   Has a large body
C   Has a greater width than the other cervical vertebrae
D   The levator scapulae muscle is attached to its transverse process
E   The odontoid process of the axis articulates with a facet in front of the posterior arch of the atlas

72 **The stapedius reflex:**
A   Loud signals presented to one ear elicit bilateral contraction of the stapedius muscle
B   The contralateral reflex usually occurs at 50–70 dB sensation level (SL) in normal ears
C   With perfect hearing, a stapedius reflex can always be induced
D   Can be used to detect non-organic hearing loss
E   The absence of a contralateral reflex with the ipsilateral reflex present may imply contralateral ossicular discontinuity

73 **The hypophysis cerebri:**
A   Weighs approximately 5 g
B   Transnasal removal is easier if the sphenoid sinus is poorly pneumatized
C   Hypophysectomy is the treatment of choice for acromegaly
D   TSH (thyroid stimulating hormone) is secreted by the acidophil cells of the pars anterior
E   The neurohypophysis is developed as a down-growth from the floor of the diencephalon

69   A F The marginal mandibular division of the facial nerve runs along the deep investing layer of fascia and may be injured if the incision is not sufficiently low.
      B F
      C T This nerve runs along the surface of the hyoglossus muscle.
      D T This is located at the uppermost surface of the gland.
      E F This nerve enters the larynx from below.

70   A F A homograft incus would come from another person or a cadaver. An autograft would be the patient's own incus.
      B F This would then be a modified radical mastoidectomy.
      C T
      D T By definition although, in a combined approach tymparoplasty, hearing restoration usually occurs in a second procedure.
      E F Disease may also be removed transcanal.

71   A F It is the first.
      B F It has no body.
      C F All except the seventh.
      D T And so are the rectus capitis lateralis, the superior and inferior obliques, splenius capitis and scalene medius.
      E F The joint is at the back of the anterior arch of the atlas.

72   A T
      B F It is usually 70–95 dB SL.
      C F The facial nerve must be functioning. Also, 5% of 'normal' ears do not have a reflex.
      D T The reflex may be elicited at a lower hearing level than the pure tone threshold.
      E T With the exception of contralateral stapedial crural discontinuity. This finding may also occur in brain stem disorders.

73   A F It weighs about 500 mg.
      B F A well-pneumatized sphenoid sinus facilitates removal. Removal may not be possible if the sinus is acellular.
      C F Bromocriptine is usually tried initially.
      D F TSH is secreted by the basophil cells of the pars anterior.
      E T

74 **Vestibular nerve section by the transtemporal (middle cranial fossa) route:**
   A   Would be performed in the presence of useful homolateral hearing
   B   Involves entering the subdural space
   C   A portion of Scarpa's ganglion should also be removed
   D   Tinnitus is controlled in almost every patient
   E   A transient facial nerve paralysis may occur postoperatively

75 **Hypersensitivity reactions:**
   A   Type 1 hypersensitivity is commonly mediated by IgE
   B   Type 2 hypersensitivity is mediated by antibodies reacting with tissue components
   C   The formation of autoantibodies against red blood cells, causing an autoimmune haemolytic anaemia, is an example of a type 3 hypersensitivity reaction
   D   Type 4 hypersensitivity depends on the formation of damaging antibody/antigen complexes
   E   The Mantoux test is an example of type 4 hypersensitivity

76 **In the larynx:**
   A   The vestibule is a fusiform recess which lies between the true and false vocal cords and may ascend lateral to the latter
   B   The lateral crico-arytenoid muscles abduct the vocal cords
   C   Mucous glands are present throughout
   D   The recurrent laryngeal nerve is motor to cricothyroid
   E   The corniculate cartilages lie in each aryepiglottic fold

77 **Hereditary causes of deafness:**
   A   Alport's syndrome has an autosomal dominant transmission
   B   Pendred's syndrome has an autosomal dominant transmission
   C   Usher's syndrome is characterized by retinitis pigmentosa and congenital sensorineural hearing loss
   D   Waardenberg's syndrome is characterized by fusion of one or more cervical vertebrae and a severe hearing loss
   E   Mondini's dysplasia is associated with musculoskeletal disease

78 **The following are characteristic of a temporal lobe abscess:**
   A   Auditory hallucinations
   B   A homonymous hemianopia
   C   Olfactory disturbances
   D   Nystagmus
   E   An intention tremor

74   A T A translabyrinthine nerve section would result in a dead ear.
      B F Surgery is entirely extradural.
      C T Thus reducing the possibility of neural regeneration.
      D F Approximately 50% notice an improvement or control of their tinnitus.
      E T Probably due to interference with its blood supply.

75   A T And is typified by acute anaphylaxis in humans.
      B T Such as the occurrence of antibodies against glomerular basement membrane in Goodpasture's syndrome.
      C F This is an example of type 2 hypersensitivity.
      D F This describes type 3 hypersensitivity.
      E T Type 4 hypersensitivity is also known as delayed-type or cell-mediated hypersensitivity.

76   A F This describes the ventricle or laryngeal sinus.
      B F They adduct the vocal cords.
      C F They are not present along the free edges of the vocal cords.
      D F It is motor to all the intrinsic laryngeal muscles except for crico-thyroid, which is supplied by the external branch of the superior laryngeal nerve.
      E F These are the cuneiform cartilages. The corniculate cartilages articulate with the summit of each arytenoid cartilage.

77   A T It is characterized by nephritis and sensorineural hearing loss.
      B F It is autosomal recessive and features a goitre and sensorineural hearing loss.
      C T It has an autosomal recessive transmission.
      D F This describes Klippel–Feil syndrome. Waardenberg's syndrome is best known for its characteristic white forelock of hair and has an autosomal dominant transmission.
      E F Mondini's dysplasia occurs without other associated anomalies.

78   A T The superior temporal gyrus represents the highest level of hearing.
      B F A quadrantic hemianopia would be more usual.
      C T Cortical olfactory centres are located in the temporal lobe.
      D F
      E F Nystagmus and an intention tremor may occur with a cerebellar abscess.

79 **Carcinoma of the bronchus:**
A   Patients may develop a painful arthropathy of the wrist, ankle and knee
B   Recurrent laryngeal nerve involvement is a sign that the tumour is incurable
C   Radiotherapy is useful palliation for haemoptysis
D   The most common site of visible or palpable lymph node enlargement is the axilla
E   The incidence of bronchial carcinoma reaches a peak in the fourth decade

80 **Laryngeal trauma:**
A   It may not be possible to visualize the vocal cords at indirect laryngoscopy following a supraglottic fracture
B   A lateral glottic fracture usually causes flattening of the prominence of the thyroid alae
C   A lateral glottic fracture will usually result in displacement of the homolateral arytenoid cartilage
D   A tracheo-oesophageal fistula may follow cricotracheal separation
E   A tracheostomy is seldom required

81 **The following are of proven value in promoting recovery of hearing for idiopathic sudden sensorineural deafness:**
A   Low molecular weight dextran
B   Prednisolone
C   Nicotinic acid
D   Cervical sympathectomy
E   Penicillin

82 **Trigeminal neuralgia:**
A   Usually begins in the third decade
B   Is more common in females
C   Eventually becomes bilateral in over 50% of cases
D   The natural history is almost always a worsening one
E   The treatment of choice is surgical

83 **Branches of the vagus nerve:**
A   The pharyngeal branch contains motor fibres to the palatoglossus muscle
B   The auricular branch carries somatic afferent nerve fibres from the mucous membrane of the middle ear
C   Oesophageal branches also supply the pericardium
D   The anterosuperior surface of the stomach is principally supplied by the left vagus nerve
E   The internal laryngeal nerve pierces the cricothyroid membrane

32   Answers

79   A T Hypertrophic pulmonary osteoarthropathy is a non-metastatic manifestation of carcinoma of the bronchus.
    B T
    C T There is an improvement of the haemoptysis in up to 95% of cases.
    D F It is the supraclavicular fossae.
    E F It peaks in the sixth decade.

80   A T Because the posteriorly displaced epiglottis and other supraglottic structures lie over the vocal cords.
    B F This occurs in a supraglottic fracture.
    C T And this prevents full glottic adduction, resulting in hoarseness.
    D T Because of associated tears in the anterior wall of the oesophagus.
    E F A tracheostomy is required in all but the least severe of cases.

81   A F Many treatments have been given, yet no single treatment has been
    B F shown to be responsible for any subsequent hearing improvement.
    C F
    D F
    E F

82   A F The majority begin in or after the fifth decade.
    B T By a 2:1 ratio.
    C F In 5% it will develop on the other side but it never starts on both sides simultaneously.
    D T
    E F It is medical, usually employing carbamazepine.

83   A T Via the pharyngeal plexus.
    B F It is sensory to a posterior section of the external auditory canal and the lateral portion of the tympanic membrane, and also a part of the cranial surface of the pinna.
    C T Its posterior aspect.
    D T And the right vagus nerve supplies its postero-inferior surface.
    E F It pierces the thyrohyoid membrane.

84   **Facial nerve paralysis:**
   A   The commonest cause of an intratemporal facial nerve paralysis is trauma
   B   Neurapraxia indicates a good prognosis for recovery
   C   A complete absence of voluntary facial movements would imply that there is a lower motor neurone lesion
   D   In the absence of facial movements, electrical tests are the only techniques available to collect objective information on the condition of the facial nerve
   E   Wallerian degeneration occurs at approximately 4–6 mm per day

85   **Epistaxis:**
   A   Kiesselbach's plexus consists only of vessels originating from the external carotid artery
   B   Seldom stops spontaneously when occurring following trauma
   C   Hypertension causes epistaxes
   D   Septal dermoplasty is of value when the cause is hereditary haemorrhagic telangiectasia
   E   Has a higher incidence in the presence of allergic rhinitis

86   **The following structures are related to the deep (medial) surface of hyoglossus:**
   A   Lingual artery
   B   Lingual nerve
   C   Glossopharyngeal nerve
   D   Hypoglossal nerve
   E   Submandibular duct

87   **Speech audiometry:**
   A   Tests the ability to hear pure tones
   B   A normal result will show a score approaching 100% at 25 dB
   C   A reversal in the direction of the curve is typical of an acoustic neuroma
   D   Patients with serous otitis media usually fail to achieve a score of 100%
   E   A shift of the normal curve to the right is seen in an acoustic neuroma

88   **Complications of total laryngectomy include:**
   A   Hypocalcaemia
   B   Pharyngeal fistula
   C   Accessory nerve paralysis
   D   Vagal nerve paralysis
   E   Chylous leak

84   A F It is idiopathic and is known as Bell's palsy.
     B T In a neurapraxic nerve there is a reversible block of impulse conduction.
     C T Some forehead movement occurs in an upper motor neurone lesion.
     D T Electroneuronography (ENoG) gives objective information on the evolution of degeneration 24 h after the onset of an intratemporal facial nerve paralysis.
     E F It has a centrifugal velocity of 4–6 cm per day, thus ENoG will usually detect degeneration within 24 h.

85   A F The anterior ethmoidal artery is derived from the internal carotid artery.
     B F Traumatic epistaxes usually cease spontaneously without treatment but severe trauma may require surgery to control the bleeding.
     C F Although there is a high incidence of epistaxes in hypertensive patients, there is little evidence that the elevated blood pressure is the cause of the bleeding.
     D T But in the long-term, the telangiectasia may recur within the skin graft.
     E T Bleeding may occur in hay fever sufferers during the pollen season if the nasal mucous membrane is severely congested.

86   A T The lingual and the hypoglossal nerves, and the submandibular duct
     B F are related to the superficial (lateral) surface of the muscle.
     C T
     D F
     E F

87   A F It assesses speech sounds.
     B F A 100% score would usually be reached at around 40 dB.
     C T
     D F There is a normal curve which is shifted to the right.
     E F Such a shift is seen most frequently in a pure conductive loss.

88   A T Despite the retention of one lobe of the thyroid, hypocalcaemia may still be a problem.
     B T A fistula is more likely to occur if the patient had previously received radiotherapy to the head and neck region.
     C F This nerve is situated out of the operative field.
     D T The vagus lies between the trachea and oesophagus, and damage may occur on separation of the two structures, although this is an extremely uncommon complication.
     E F The thoracic duct should not be exposed unless the operation is accompanied by a neck dissection.

89 **Peptic ulceration:**
    A   Occurs only in the oesophagus, stomach or duodenum
    B   Cimetidine is an H_2 receptor agonist
    C   A posterior duodenal ulcer would be more likely to perforate than would an anterior duodenal ulcer
    D   Antacids are chemicals that neutralize the hydrochloric acid secreted by the gastric parietal cells
    E   A typical benign gastric ulcer occurs on or near the greater curvature

90 **Dural venous sinuses:**
    A   The superior sagittal sinus occupies the attached convex margin of the falx cerebri
    B   The left transverse sinus is usually a direct continuation of the superior sagittal sinus
    C   The superior sagittal sinus receives the great cerebral vein
    D   The inferior petrosal sinuses drain the cavernous sinus into the sigmoid sinuses
    E   The superior petrosal sinuses drain the cavernous sinus into the sigmoid sinuses

91 **Tympanic membrane perforations:**
    A   Are usually multiple when caused by tuberculosis
    B   Of the pars flaccida are associated with cholesteatoma
    C   Following acute otitis media will usually heal spontaneously
    D   Commonly occur following transverse fractures of the petrous temporal bone
    E   Are always associated with a conductive deafness

92 **Salivary glands:**
    A   The secretions of the sublingual gland are chiefly mucoid
    B   The secretions of the parotid gland are chiefly serous
    C   The lingual nerve carries secretomotor fibres to the submandibular gland
    D   The parotid gland is directly related to the medial pterygoid muscle
    E   The parotid duct opens opposite the lower second molar tooth

93 **Advantages of 'canal wall up' over 'canal wall down' otologic procedures:**
    A   An anatomically normal ear is restored
    B   Later ossicular reconstruction is a more feasible proposition
    C   An open mastoid cavity is avoided
    D   There is less risk of damaging the facial nerve
    E   The incidence of residual cholesteatoma is lower

89　A　F　It may also occur at the site of anastomosis of a gastroenterostomy or in a Meckel's diverticulum.
　　B　F　It is an H_2 receptor antagonist.
　　C　F　The converse is true. A posterior duodenal ulcer would be more likely to bleed.
　　D　T
　　E　F　It occurs on or near the lesser curvature of the stomach.

90　A　T
　　B　F　It is usually the right transverse sinus.
　　C　F　The straight sinus receives the great cerebral vein.
　　D　F　They drain them into the internal jugular vein.
　　E　F　They drain them into the transverse sinuses.

91　A　T
　　B　T　As are posteromarginal perforations of the pars tensa.
　　C　T　The tympanic membrane will usually adopt its normal appearance within 2–3 weeks.
　　D　F　However, they may occur following longitudinal fractures.
　　E　F　There may be normal hearing when the perforation is small, especially if it is anterior.

92　A　T
　　B　T
　　C　T　Courtesy of the chorda tympani nerve.
　　D　T　And anteriorly it also impinges on the masseter.
　　E　F　It opens opposite the upper second molar.

93　A　T
　　B　T　Because the ear is more anatomically normal.
　　C　T
　　D　F　Although uncommon in experienced hands, there is a higher risk of a facial nerve paralysis in a 'canal wall up' procedure.
　　E　F　It is higher since visibility and access of most middle ear areas is poorer, e.g. the sinus tympani.

94 **The oropharynx contains the following areas:**
  A The valleculae
  B The hard palate
  C The superior surface of the uvula
  D The inferior surface of the uvula
  E The laryngeal (posterior) surface of the epiglottis

95 **'Malignant' otitis externa:**
  A Is a disorder of viral aetiology
  B Is more common in diabetics
  C Antibiotic therapy should be withheld until the affecting
     organism has been isolated and its sensitivity is known
  D May rapidly spread to affect the skull-base
  E Surgical treatment is always indicated

96 **The sternocleidomastoid muscle:**
  A Is a boundary of the anterior triangle of the neck
  B Is a boundary of the posterior triangle of the neck
  C Derives its nerve supply exclusively from the accessory nerve
  D Inserts into the superior nuchal line superiorly
  E Is deep to platysma

97 **Nasal packs:**
  A A posterior nasal pack should contain at least three tapes
  B Anterior nasal packs must be removed within 48 h of insertion
  C Antibiotic therapy should be instituted if a posterior nasal pack
     remains *in situ* for more than 24 h
  D Should always be inserted under a general anaesthetic
  E May result in mental disturbances

98 **The auricle:**
  A Its curved prominent rim is called the helix
  B The scaphoid fossa is formed by the division of the antihelix into
     two crura
  C Is composed of a thin plate of hyaline cartilage
  D The antitragus lies below the crus of the helix and in front of the
     concha
  E Its skin is continuous with that of the external auditory canal

99 **The inner ear fluids:**
  A The scala vestibuli contains endolymph
  B Endolymph has a similar chemical composition to other
     extracellular fluids
  C Perilymph has a similar chemical composition to other
     extracellular fluids
  D Are thought to be reabsorbed within the endolymphatic sac
  E Communicate with the subarachnoid space

94   A T
      B F The oropharynx extends from the junction of the hard and the soft palate.
      C F This is a part of the floor of the nasopharynx.
      D T
      E F But the anterior (lingual) surface is included.

95   A F The usual organism is the bacterium *Pseudomonas aeruginosa.*
      B T It occurs more usually in elderly diabetics.
      C F Prompt diagnosis and treatment is essential since there is up to 80% mortality once cranial nerve involvement has occurred.
      D T And may involve the jugular foramen, including the last four cranial nerves, and the infratemporal fossa.
      E F The treatment of choice is prolonged medical therapy. Surgery is of secondary importance and usually consists of ear canal debridement and removal of granulation tissue, but this is not always necessary.

96   A T Its anterior border forms the posterior boundary of the anterior triangle.
      B T Its posterior border forms the anterior border of the posterior triangle.
      C F Ventral rami of the second, third and fourth cervical nerves are proprioceptive to the muscle and possibly also motor.
      D T And also into the lateral surface of the mastoid process.
      E T

97   A T Such that the pack is secured in front of the nostril by tying together two nasal tapes over a bolster, and a tape exiting through the mouth is required as an aid for removal of the pack.
      B F They may remain for over a week but antibiotic therapy would be required for packs remaining *in situ* for longer than 48 h.
      C F Antibiotic therapy should be commenced as soon as the pack is inserted.
      D F Although this would be preferable for children, topical anaesthesia is usually sufficient for adults.
      E T Confusion may occur in the elderly due to increased hypoxia caused by the presence of the pack and also due to stasis and sepsis behind a pack.

98   A T
      B F This describes the triangular fossa.
      C F It is composed of a thin layer of fibrocartilage.
      D F This is the tragus.
      E T

99   A F It contains perilymph, as does the scala tympani.
      B F It is the only extracellular fluid in the body with a high potassium ion content.
      C T
      D T Problems in this mechanism are thought to play a role in the aetiology of Menière's disease.
      E T Via the aqueduct of the cochlea.

100 **Lasers in otolaryngology:**
    A   The word LASER is an acronym
    B   The most effective laser in the management of vascular lesions is the argon laser
    C   Complications of carbon dioxide laser endoscopy include endotracheal tube fires
    D   The argon laser can be used to perform stapedectomy
    E   The carbon dioxide laser can transmit through flexible bundles

101 **The forehead flap:**
    A   Derives its blood supply from the supra-orbital and supratrochlear branches of the internal carotid artery, and the frontal branches of the superficial temporal artery from the external carotid artery
    B   Would be useful for creating a new hypopharynx
    C   Is well suited to repair a defect in the floor of the mouth
    D   There is an obvious cosmetic defect even after the donor site has healed
    E   The cosmetic defect is more acceptable if the unused part of the flap is not returned

102 **Myringotomy:**
    A   The function of a ventilating tube is to allow the drainage of middle ear fluid
    B   Would be indicated in acute suppurative otitis media with a bulging tympanic membrane
    C   The usual site of incision in the tympanic membrane is the anterior and inferior segment
    D   On average, a simple grommet will stay in place for 18 months
    E   There is a risk of damage to the jugular bulb

103 **Multiple sclerosis:**
    A   There is an increased risk of acquiring the disease if there is a positive family history
    B   Brain stem lesions are common and early
    C   The age of onset is usually between 40 and 60 years
    D   Progresses steadily
    E   Is thought to be caused by a bacterium

104 **The thoracic duct:**
    A   Begins around the twelfth thoracic vertebra
    B   Opens into the junction of the left internal jugular vein and left brachiocephalic vein
    C   Contains no valves
    D   Descends in front of the second part of the subclavian artery prior to its termination
    E   Passes anterior to the phrenic nerve

40   Answers

100 A T It means 'Light Amplification by Stimulated Emission of Radiation'.
     B T Because of its inherent affinity for haemoglobin.
     C T If the tube is unprotected or its coverings are dehiscent.
     D T Although there is doubt about its advantages over conventional surgical techniques.
     E F This is only possible with the argon laser and the Nd (neodymium)–YAG (yttrium aluminium garnet) laser.

101 A T
     B F It is not long enough.
     C T And other deficiencies above this level.
     D T Therefore other types of flap will often be preferred.
     E T The defect although larger if the remainder of the flap is not returned, is symmetrical and therefore less conspicuous.

102 A F It is to establish adequate aeration of the middle ear cleft.
     B T But the most common indication is secretory otitis media.
     C T Here there is less chance of damage to many of the important structures of the middle ear, most of which lie posteriorly and superiorly.
     D F It is usually 6–9 months, unless a ventilation tube is inserted with the specific purpose of long-term aeration (T-tube).
     E T Occasionally the jugular bulb is situated in the lower mesotympanum.

103 A T A relative of the patient with the disease has a risk 15–25 times that in the general population.
     B T And include diplopia, vertigo and facial weakness as presenting features.
     C F It is 20–40 years.
     D F It is characterized by multiple exacerbations and remissions but in the later stages relapses heal incompletely, contributing to the progressive disability.
     E F Although the pathogenesis is unknown, recent interest centres around a slow virus or an autoimmune process.

104 A T At the upper end of the cisterna chyli.
     B F It opens into the junction of the left internal jugular vein and the left subclavian vein.
     C F There are several valves which correspond to the sites of exposure to pressure.
     D F It is the first part.
     E T It is separated from it by the prevertebral fascia.

105 **Cholesteatoma:**
  A   A primary (congenital) cholesteatoma may arise as an ingrowth of keratinizing stratified squamous epithelium from the edge of a tympanic membrane perforation, or secondarily to a tympanic membrane retraction
  B   Primary (congenital) cholesteatoma usually always manifests itself in the first two decades of life
  C   Induces resorption of underlying bone
  D   May become manifest by the presentation of meningitis
  E   May develop following a fracture of the temporal bone

106 **Features of hypothyroidism include:**
  A   Goitre
  B   Hoarseness
  C   Deafness
  D   Nasal obstruction
  E   Enlarged tongue

107 **Vertebrobasilar ischaemia:**
  A   Is the cause of 20% of all cerebrovascular accidents
  B   May produce occipital lobe dysfunction
  C   The posterior cerebral arteries are the terminal branches of the basilar artery
  D   Symptoms may be confined to a specific cranial nerve
  E   Hyperextension with rotation of the head and neck can reduce blood flow in one or both vertebral arteries

108 **Development of the thyroid gland:**
  A   The thyroglossal duct may persist as an epithelial tract
  B   The thyroglossal duct may persist as a series of blind pockets
  C   The pyramidal lobe is an outgrowth from the left lobe of the thyroid
  D   The pyramidal lobe is more prominent in adults than children
  E   Complete congenital absence of the thyroid gland is seldom noticed until a few weeks after birth

109 **Oesophageal foreign bodies:**
  A   Occur more frequently in those people wearing dentures
  B   The best investigation for detection is a chest X-ray
  C   Impact randomly along the oesophagus
  D   Are generally most successfully removed using a flexible fibreoptic oesophagogastroscope
  E   Following the ingestion of too large a foreign body, an early symptom is a sensation of choking or gagging

42   Answers

105   A   F   These are the commoner causes of a secondary (acquired) cholesteatoma.

    B   F   Only for those cholesteatomas of the middle ear and mastoid. Those at the petrous apex usually become evident between 35 and 55 years of age.

    C   T   Possibly by means of collagenolytic and other enzymes.

    D   T   Although the more usual presenting features are deafness and aural discharge.

    E   T   As a consequence of implantation of keratinizing squamous epithelium through the fracture line.

106   A   T   Especially in Hashimoto's disease, dyshormonogenesis, following the administration of certain drugs, and in iodine deficient areas.

    B   T   The voice is low pitched and speech slow.

    C   T   This is usually a high frequency sensorineural hearing loss.

    D   T   Hypothyroidism is one of the endocrine diseases that affects the nose.

    E   T

107   A   T

    B   T   And also dysfunction of the brain stem and the cerebellar hemispheres.

    C   T   And the basilar artery is the union of the two vertebral arteries.

    D   T   But other abnormalities in the structures supplied by the vertebrobasilar system usually become manifest in ensuing weeks.

    E   T   The second to seventh cervical vertebrae possess their own canals for the vertebral vessels.

108   A   T   It would then remain open from the foramen caecum of the tongue to the level of the larynx.

    B   T   These are thyroglossal duct cysts.

    C   F   It results from the retention and growth of the lower end of the thyroglossal duct.

    D   F   The converse is true since it undergoes progressive atrophy.

    E   T   The fetus is supplied with sufficient maternal thyroid hormone to permit normal development.

109   A   T   Coverage of the roof of the mouth by dentures decreases palatal sensation and thus prevents certain foreign bodies from being detected.

    B   F   A lateral neck X-ray is the most useful investigation.

    C   F   There are 3 principal sites where foreign bodies tend to lodge and these are at 15, 24 and 40 cm from the incisor teeth.

    D   F   A rigid pharyngoscope or oesophagoscope usually allows for a more successful removal.

    E   T   Followed by dysphagia, drooling of saliva and retrosternal pain.

110 **Following a rhinoplasty:**
   A   Secondary surgery should not be performed until 3 months
   B   The most common early postoperative complication is infection
   C   Transient epiphora may occur
   D   Patients may develop a persistent obstructive vasomotor type of rhinitis
   E   Columellar retraction may occur following resection of the membranous septum

111 **ENT head mirrors in common usage:**
   A   Most have a diameter of $3\frac{1}{2}$ inches
   B   The central aperture is $1\frac{1}{4}$ inches
   C   The mirror is convex
   D   The source of light should be concentrated at a focal length of 12 inches
   E   ENT visualization should ideally be only via the eye looking through the central aperture

112 **Patient selection for stapedectomy:**
   A   The incidence of failure is higher in patients under 20 years of age
   B   A moderate to severe homolateral mixed sensorineural hearing loss is a contraindication for surgery
   C   Unilateral hearing loss only is a contraindication for surgery
   D   In bilateral disease, surgery would usually be performed on the worse hearing ear
   E   A positive Schwartze sign is not a contraindication to surgery

113 **Industrial noise-induced hearing loss:**
   A   May feature a 6 kHz 'notch' on a pure tone audiogram
   B   Is usually characterized by recruitment of loudness
   C   There is no direct relationship between the extent of the hearing loss and the noise exposure
   D   Tinnitus is slowly progressive over many years
   E   Otorrhoea is present in approximately 50% of patients

114 **When considering middle ear surgery performed under local anaesthesia (LA):**
   A   Intra-operative bleeding is less than under general anaesthesia
   B   A postoperative facial paralysis may occur
   C   The patient is never aware of manipulations around the vestibule
   D   Revision surgery usually requires the use of a greater volume of LA solution
   E   The addition of a vasoconstrictor to the LA solution is unnecessary

44   Answers

110   A F It should not be performed for at least 6–12 months. The nose changes continually after surgery and oedema may persist for long periods.
      B F This is surprisingly rare. Haemorrhage is more common..
      C T Because of the proximity of the lacrimal apparatus to the lateral osteotomy site.
      D T In approximately 10% of patients there is a persistent postoperative enlargement of the inferior turbinates, which may be alleviated by the use of topical intranasal steroids.
      E T But it also occurs with the excessive removal of the inferior caudal margin of the nasal septum, resulting in cicatrization.

111   A T
      B F It is 3/4 inch.
      C F It is concave.
      D F It should be nearer 8 inches.
      E F Visualization is binocular.

112   A T Due to the activity of the otosclerotic growth, which is probably stimulated by the surgery.
      B F Hearing improvement may be sufficient to allow for more effective use of amplification.
      C F It is not contraindicated but most UK surgeons will not perform the operation in the presence of normal contralateral hearing.
      D T Lest a complete sensorineural deafness should result from the surgery.
      E T Increased vascularization of the mucous membrane over the promontory is visualized as a reddish glow through the tympanic membrane, and probably indicates otosclerotic activity. Most surgeons feel that this alone is not a surgical contraindication.

113   A T But the presence of a 4 kHz 'notch' is more common.
      B T There is usually cochlear, rather than neural, damage.
      C F There is invariably a relationship between the two but the sensitivity of individuals to noise varies greatly.
      D T This is quite common.
      E F Otorrhoea is not associated with industrial noise-induced hearing loss.

114   A T Even without the use of a vasoconstrictor agent.
      B T The LA may affect the tympanic part of the facial nerve if there is a bony dehiscence or the main trunk may be affected by periauricular injections and the paresis will be transient.
      C F The patient may complain of vertigo, especially during revision surgery.
      D T Due to the presence of scars and adhesions limiting the distribution of the LA to the nearby tissues.
      E F Bleeding is reduced.

115 **Olfaction:**
   A   Parosmia implies normality
   B   Part of the olfactory organ is located in the nasal septum
   C   Hyposmia is a reduced sensation of olfaction
   D   A grossly deviated nasal septum may cause a complete loss of olfaction
   E   Influenza may produce anosmia

116 **Glomus jugulare tumours:**
   A   Arise from chemoreceptor tissue situated along the vagus nerve
   B   Are usually malignant
   C   Carotid angiography is essential
   D   Involvement by the tumour of the vagus, the accessory and the hypoglossal nerves, but not the glossopharyngeal nerve, constitutes Vernet's syndrome
   E   As a consequence of the tumour, patients may have evidence of middle ear involvement

117 **Blood transfusion:**
   A   An autologous blood transfusion is one where the donor is a blood relative of the recipient
   B   In an emergency, a patient with a blood group of O rhesus negative would usually be considered a universal recipient
   C   Malaria may be transmitted in contaminated blood
   D   An average male will have a circulating blood volume of 50 ml/kg
   E   Blood intended for transfusion may be stored for up to 2 months

118 **Maxillary sinus lavage:**
   A   When checking the instruments, the tip of the trocar should ideally be at the level of the distal part of the cannula when fully inserted
   B   Is indicated in suspected cases of maxillary sinus neoplasms
   C   Should be performed in children under 3 years with suspected sinus disease
   D   Is usually performed under general anaesthesia
   E   No serious complications can occur

119 **Ludwig's angina:**
   A   Consists of pain in the tongue on movement
   B   Its incidence is increased in the presence of dental disease
   C   Treatment is by surgical drainage
   D   Respiratory obstruction may occur
   E   The usual organism is *Streptococcus pyogenes*

46 Answers

115 A F It refers to a distortion of the sense of smell.
  B T The specialized neuroepithelium is also located above and in the region of the superior turbinate and in the nasal roof at the level of the cribriform plate.
  C T
  D T This would be most unusual, but may occur in complete obstruction although there may be hyposmia in partial obstruction.
  E T And also other cranial nerve neuropathies, especially of the facial and vagus nerves.

116 A F They arise from chemoreceptor tissue in the area of the jugular bulb.
  B F This would be exceptional.
  C T The extent of the vascularity of the tumour and its dimensions are demonstrated. A computerized tomographic (CT) scan is also essential.
  D F This would be Jackson's syndrome. Vernet's syndrome affects the glossopharyngeal, vagus and accessory nerves, and spares the hypoglossal nerve. If the latter also becomes involved, a Collet-Sicard syndrome would be present.
  E T Conductive deafness, pulsatile tinnitus and otalgia are common.

117 A F It is one in which the recipient has previously been the donor of the blood.
  B F This patient would be a universal donor. A universal recipient would have the group AB rhesus (+).
  C T Other transmissible infections include syphilis, hepatitis, cytomegalovirus and AIDS.
  D F It is 75 ml/kg.
  E F 21 days is the usual limit.

118 A F It should project approximately 3 mm beyond the cannula.
  B F A biopsy should be carried out, preferably via an intranasal antrostomy.
  C F The sinus may be so small that attempted lavage is dangerous.
  D F This is usual only in children and in adults in whom it is incidental to other procedures.
  E F The orbit may be penetrated and the optic nerve damaged.

119 A F It is a spreading cellulitis of the floor of the mouth and submandibular space.
  B T Over 80% of patients have severe dental disease.
  C F Pus is seldom found and treatment is by antibiotics.
  D T Because the tongue is elevated posterosuperiorly.
  E F It is commonly *Streptococcus viridans* or *Escherichia coli*.

120 **Hearing aids (excluding cochlear implants):**
   A   There is usually more benefit obtained when the hearing loss is conductive rather than sensorineural
   B   Are of little benefit for a unilateral hearing loss
   C   Are very helpful when there is difficulty in speech discrimination
   D   The only disadvantage of a 'body worn' aid is its appearance
   E   A bone conduction aid is most useful in the presence of a severe or profound hearing loss

121 **Squamous carcinoma of the larynx:**
   A   Glottic lesions most frequently present with throat discomfort
   B   Subglottic lesions most frequently present with stridor
   C   Supraglottic lesions account for approximately 20% of all laryngeal neoplasms
   D   The most frequent supraglottic site is the suprahyoid epiglottis
   E   Is associated with carcinoma of the bronchus

122 **Features of meningitis include:**
   A   Otorrhoea
   B   Photophilia
   C   Fluctuating pyrexia
   D   Headache
   E   *Haemophilus influenzae* as the infecting agent in young adults

123 **Veins of the head and neck:**
   A   The pterygoid plexus lies around and within the lateral pterygoid muscle
   B   The facial vein is formed from the junction of the supratrochlear and supra-orbital veins
   C   The posterior branch of the retromandibular vein joins the posterior auricular vein to form the external jugular vein
   D   The pterygoid plexus communicates with the cavernous sinus
   E   The internal jugular vein is a direct continuation of the sigmoid sinus

124 **Tuberculosis:**
   A   Responsible organisms may be seen on a smear using the Lowenstein–Jensen stain
   B   Droplet spread is the commonest mode of transmission
   C   A 'Ghon' lesion is active
   D   Miliary tuberculosis occurs when there is unchecked haematogenous spread
   E   Caseation refers to necrosis within the area of inflammation

48 Answers

120 A T Because the fault is in amplification rather than sound processing.
   B T The normal ear will usually compensate well for the loss.
   C F They may amplify the sound but the problem of discrimination is not solved.
   D F Other disadvantages are noise resulting from the aid rubbing against the clothes and lack of directional information.
   E F It would be used when there is an actively discharging ear, which would preclude the use of an ear mould, or other contraindications to putting an ear mould in the caral.

121 A F They usually present with hoarseness.
   B T
   C F It is nearer 40%. Glottic lesions account for 55% and subglottic lesions for 5%.
   D F It is the infrahyoid epiglottis.
   E T Any patient with a carcinoma of the upper air and food passages has an increased incidence of developing a second neoplasm in this area and also in the bronchi.

122 A F Although suppurative otitis media may be the cause of the meningitis.
   B F Photophobia is common.
   C F A fluctuating pyrexia is a prominent feature of a sigmoid sinus thrombosis, which is unlike that of meningitis.
   D T This is often the most frequent and significant initial complaint.
   E F This organism causes meningitis in infants and young children.

123 A T
   B T And as the common facial vein it drains into the internal jugular vein.
   C T It empties into the subclavian vein.
   D T Usually through the foramen ovale.
   E T It then joins with the subclavian vein to form the brachiocephalic vein.

124 A F This is culture medium. The smear would be stained by the Ziehl–Neelson method.
   B T Although tubercle bacilli may enter the gastrointestinal tract from infected milk, from swallowing infected expectorated sputum or through contact with injured skin or mucous membranes.
   C F A 'Ghon' lesion represents the primary pulmonary focus which has healed to a fibrosed and calcific lesion and, in time, the lymph nodes regress and calcify.
   D T This can occur in the absence of adequate immunity and may result in meningitis or scattered small lesions throughout the lung fields.
   E T The term caseation is used because the gross appearance is cheesy.

125 **The nerve supply of the soft palate:**
- A   Tensor palati is supplied by the pharyngeal plexus
- B   Levator palati is supplied by the pharyngeal plexus
- C   Palatoglossus is supplied by the hypoglossal nerve
- D   The pharyngeal branch of the sphenopalatine ganglion is sensory to its upper surface
- E   Its taste buds are supplied by the greater (superficial) petrosal nerve

126 **Injury to the cervical spine:**
- A   The Brown–Séquard syndrome represents the consequence of complete spinal cord transection
- B   Flexion injuries usually occur following forceful deceleration in a motor vehicle
- C   A 'hangman's' fracture is a flexion–rotation injury
- D   Compression injuries are the commonest
- E   Respiratory embarrassment may occur following spinal cord transection below the level of the sixth cervical vertebra

127 **The facial nerve:**
- A   Is entirely motor
- B   Is motor to stylohyoid
- C   Its intracranial portion is supplied by the anterior inferior cerebellar artery
- D   The narrowest part of the fallopian canal is at the junction of the meatal and labyrinthine segments
- E   Its tympanic segment lies inferior to the cochleariform process

128 **The superior orbital fissure:**
- A   Is bounded superiorly by the lesser wing of the sphenoid
- B   Is a continuation of the pterygopalatine and infratemporal fossae
- C   Transmits the optic nerve
- D   The nasociliary nerve is lateral to the abducent nerve
- E   The trochlear nerve remains outside the cone of muscles

129 **Cerebrospinal fluid:**
- A   Is reabsorbed into the blood by the choroid plexuses
- B   Approximately 450 ml is produced each day
- C   Flows from the third to the fourth ventricle via the cerebral aqueduct of Sylvius
- D   Flows from the lateral ventricles to the third ventricle via the foramina of Magendie
- E   Circulates as far as the level of the second sacral vertebra

125   A F It is supplied from the motor division of the trigeminal nerve.
      B T From accessory nerve fibres carried in the pharyngeal branch of the vagus.
      C F It is supplied from the pharyngeal plexus.
      D T After having passed through the palatovaginal canal.
      E T The cell bodies are in the geniculate ganglion.

126   A F It represents the consequence of hemisection.
      B T Or from a blow to the back of the head.
      C F It is a hyperextension injury.
      D F They are uncommon because during the injury the spine would need to be perfectly straight.
      E T Because of loss of intercostal function. The phrenic nerve, however, will still be functioning normally.

127   A F It is sensory to a poorly-specified area of the skin of the external auditory meatus.
      B T And also to stapedius, the posterior belly of digastric and the muscles of facial expression.
      C T
      D T It is no greater than 0.68 mm here and may account for the site of pathology in Bell's palsy.
      E F It is superior.

128   A T The greater wing of the sphenoid is inferior, the body of the sphenoid is medial and the frontal bone is lateral.
      B F This is the inferior orbital fissure.
      C F The optic nerve passes through the optic foramen.
      D T
      E T Along with the lacrimal and frontal nerves.

129   A F This is its origin. It is reabsorbed into the blood through the arachnoid villi (granulations).
      B T
      C T
      D F It is via the interventricular foramen of Monro.
      E T The subarachnoid space extends this far.

130 **Aural syringing:**

A An ear should not be syringed unless the tympanic membrane is thought to be intact

B The best irrigating solution is tap water at room temperature

C During the procedure the patient may develop a bradycardia

D The water should be squirted directly at the wax

E In order to straighten the external auditory canal prior to syringing, the pinna should be gently retracted in a downwards and backwards direction

131 **The Rinne test:**

A Is positive when the sound perceived by the patient is louder by air conduction than by bone conduction

B A positive Rinne implies normal hearing in that ear

C Becomes negative when there is a conductive deafness greater than 15–20 dB

D A unilateral total deafness may show a Rinne negative response

E For accurate diagnosis, the Rinne test should only be analysed in conjunction with the Weber test

132 **Viral hepatitis:**

A Hepatitis A is more commonly spread by the faeco-oral route

B In the UK the incidence of carriers of hepatitis B virus is approximately 1%

C Non-A non-B hepatitis is generally mild

D Hepatitis B has an incubation period of between 2 and 5 months

E In hepatitis A the virus is excreted in the faeces only *after* the onset of jaundice

133 **The maxillary sinus:**

A Is a pyramidal cavity in the body of the maxilla

B Drains into the nose via one ostium

C Its floor is lower than the floor of the nasal cavity

D The infra-orbital nerve usually projects into the sinus

E Lies entirely within the maxilla

134 **Menière's disease:**

A Prosper Menière published his papers early in the twentieth century

B Is characterized by a persistent and progressive sensorineural hearing loss

C Tinnitus is invariably pulsatile

D Vestibular nerve section by the transtemporal (middle cranial fossa) route preserves hearing

E The endolymphatic spaces are distended

52   Answers

130 A T Otherwise the irrigating solution may damage a weakened tympanic membrane or enter the middle ear through a perforation which is already present.
     B F The correct temperature is 37°C (body temperature). Saline would be safer than tap water if a perforation does exist.
     C T Due to the stimulation of the auricular branch of the vagus.
     D F If this were the case, the wax would be pushed further medially. Ideally, the stream should be directed towards the canal roof or aimed between the tympanic membrane and the wax.
     E F It should be retracted upwards and backwards.

131 A T And vice versa.
     B F It implies only a normal sound conducting mechanism.
     C T But the Weber test may localize with a 5 dB difference between the two ears.
     D T Termed a 'false-negative' Rinne response, it occurs because the sound transmitted by bone conduction is perceived in the good ear.
     E T Otherwise diagnostic errors may occur.

132 A T And hepatitis B is usually spread by parenteral transmission.
     B F It is 0.1%.
     C T Except in pregnant women, where fulminant hepatitis may frequently develop.
     D T Hepatitis A has an incubation period of 2–6 weeks.
     E F It is excreted in the faeces for about 2 weeks *before* the onset of jaundice but for only a few days *after* the development of symptoms.

133 A T
     B F There may be a second, smaller, accessory ostium, which also opens into the middle meatus.
     C T Its lowest part may be 1.25 cm lower than the nasal floor.
     D T This well-marked ridge extends along the roof to the anterior wall.
     E F Its medial boundary also consists of the inferior turbinate and parts of the etumoid and palatine bones.

134 A F They were published in 1861.
     B F The hearing loss is characteristically fluctuant.
     C F It is usually non-pulsatile.
     D T All hearing is destroyed following vestibular nerve section by the translabyrinthine route.
     E T This is the rationale for endolymphatic sac surgery.

135 **Nasal polyps:**
  A   Are benign neoplasms
  B   Typically occur in allergic rhinitis
  C   May resolve on treatment with topical nasal steroids
  D   Usually arise from the maxillary sinus
  E   Are more common in those over 30 years of age

136 **Laryngocoeles:**
  A   Arise from the saccule of the laryngeal ventricle
  B   Usually pass through the thyrohyoid membrane and present as a
       mass in the neck
  C   Are occupationally related
  D   Increase in size when the Valsalva manoeuvre is performed
  E   May result in airway obstruction

137 **Cleft palate:**
  A   Occurs in approximately 1 in 5000 Caucasian births
  B   Is familial
  C   A submucous cleft of the soft palate is associated with a bifid
       uvula
  D   Is associated with deafness
  E   Speech is hyponasal

138 **ENT journals:**
  A   *Acta Otolaryngologica* is published in the USA
  B   *Clinical Otolaryngology* is published every other month
  C   The *Journal of Laryngology and Otology* has been published for
       over 100 years
  D   *Clinical Otolaryngology* has been published only since 1976
  E   *Archives of Otolaryngology* is the official publication of the
       American Academy of Facial, Plastic and Reconstructive Surgery

139 **The palatine tonsil:**
  A   Is situated between the palatoglossal arch anteriorly and the
       palatopharyngeal arch posteriorly
  B   Its medial surface has 12–15 orifices
  C   Is medial to the superior constrictor muscle
  D   Its principal blood supply is derived from the tonsillar branch of
       the facial artery
  E   Its sensation is derived from the lingual nerve

140 **Keratosis obturans:**
  A   A cholesteatoma-like mass fills the external auditory meatus
  B   Is associated with thyrotoxicosis
  C   Is associated with the development of squamous cell carcinoma
  D   Surgical treatment includes a mastoidectomy
  E   Is associated with chronic sinusitis

135   A F Nasal polyps are formed from oedematous and inflamed nasal submucosa.
B F They occur in the eosinophilic variant of vasomotor rhinitis and are no more common in other nasal conditions than would be expected by chance.
C T Polyps regress with steroids, which are very effective for treating eosinophilic vasomotor rhinitis.
D F They usually arise from within the ethmoidal sinuses but the middle turbinate can become polypoidal. Antrochoanal polypi do arise from the maxillary sinus.
E T Nasal polyposis is rare below 30 years of age and cystic fibrosis should be suspected when the polyps occur in children.

136   A T They are epithelial-lined diverticula.
B F Only the external laryngocele does this.
C T There is an increased incidence in glass blowers and in wind instrument musicians.
D T There is an increase in the intraluminal pressure of the laryngocele.
E T An internal laryngocele may displace and enlarge the false vocal cord but rarely causes stridor.

137   A F Its incidence is approximately 1 in 750.
B T The tendency towards cleft palate formation does tend to run in families.
C T A bifid uvula is the mildest form of cleft palate.
D T Such patients often have glue ear because of the associated eustachian tube dysfunction.
E F It is hypernasal because of the excessive emission of air through the nose.

138   A F It is a Swedish publication.
B T
C T Its centenary was celebrated in 1985.
D T
E T And also of the American Society of Head and Neck Surgery.

139   A T These are the anterior and posterior pillars of the fauces.
B T Which lead into the tonsillar crypts.
C T And to the styloglossus muscle.
D T Although it also receives blood from the lingual, ascending pharyngeal and maxillary arteries.
E F It is principally from the glossopharyngeal nerve with additional branches from the lesser palatine nerve.

140   A T Usually, only the deep meatus is affected while the cartilaginous meatus is not involved.
B F
C T This has occasionally been observed.
D F Removal of the mass is usually all that is required.
E T And also bronchiectasis.

141 **Carcinoma of the tongue:**
  A   Frequently causes a hypoglossal nerve paralysis
  B   Commonly occurs over its dorsum
  C   May present with otalgia
  D   Syphilis is a predisposing factor
  E   Is $1\frac{1}{2}$ times more common in the anterior two thirds compared to the posterior third

142 **Hypertension:**
  A   Essential hypertension is usually due to renal disease
  B   Phaeochromocytoma is associated with rapid fluctuations in blood pressure
  C   Causes epistaxes
  D   Is often symptomless
  E   In most cases there is no known cause

143 **Allergy to fungal spores:**
  A   Is a moderately important cause of allergic rhinitis in summer
  B   Is easily diagnosed by RAST testing
  C   Is easily diagnosed by challenge testing
  D   *Cladosporium herbarum* is the most important fungus causing allergic symptoms
  E   The important allergens are those fungal spores occurring most commonly in the atmosphere

144 **The anterior cervical triangle:**
  A   Is bounded posteriorly by the posterior border of sternomastoid
  B   The submental triangle contains the submandibular gland
  C   The carotid triangle contains the vagus nerve
  D   The digastric triangle is bounded superiorly by the base of the mandible
  E   Has its apex at the sternum

145 **Surgical approaches to the middle ear and mastoid:**
  A   A posterior tympanotomy affords good access to the facial recess
  B   A postaural incision is chosen for a translabyrinthine approach to the internal auditory meatus
  C   An endaural incision has no disadvantages
  D   A permeatal incision is useful in the presence of external otitis
  E   Stapedectomy may be performed via an endaural incision

146 **Total laryngectomy:**
  A   The patient should be in the 'sniffing the morning air' position
  B   The hyoid bone is always removed
  C   A Gluck–Sorensen incision is preferred in the irradiated patient
  D   The strap muscles are divided at their superior attachment
  E   The trachea is divided at the level of the second tracheal ring

141   A   F This would be most unusual.
      B   F The lateral lingual border is the most frequent site of occurrence (85–90%).
      C   T The pain is referred.
      D   F Although syphilis has been described as being a risk factor, there is little evidence to support this view.
      E   F It is approximately five times more common.

142   A   F It is idiopathic.
      B   T This is typical.
      C   F Although the two are associated.
      D   T The great majority of patients are symptomless, even those with severe hypertension. Hypertension is usually discovered on routine examination or when complications have occurred.
      E   T In approximately 90% of cases the hypertension is essential (idiopathic, primary).

143   A   T It is probable that fungal spores are a common cause of rhinitis and asthma but the diagnosis is difficult.
      B   F RAST correlates poorly with clinical fungal allergy.
      C   F Challenge testing is also a poor correlator.
      D   T This is the most common airborne fungal spore.
      E   T The most important fungal allergens are those that occur in the greatest frequency and in descending order of importance they are *Cladosporium, Alternaria, Aspergillus* and *Penicillium*.

144   A   F Its posterior border is the anterior border of sternomastoid.
      B   F This is situated in the digastric triangle.
      C   F This nerve is excluded from the carotid triangle as it lies entirely subjacent to the sternomastoid muscle.
      D   T And also by a line drawn from the angle of the mandible to the mastoid process.
      E   T The anterior triangle is subdivided into the muscular, carotid, digastric and submental triangles.

145   A   T Because it opens lateral to two vertical segment of the facial nerve.
      B   T
      C   F Stenosis may occur at the bony/cartilaginous junction and access to the mastoid tip cells may be difficult.
      D   F This is a contraindication.
      E   T Especially in the presence of a narrow external auditory canal.

146   A   F Both the cervical spine and the atlanto-occipital joint should be extended.
      B   T To ensure clearance of the pre-epiglottic space.
      C   F A double-horizontal Mcfee incision would be more advisable.
      D   F They are divided inferiorly.
      E   F There is no strict rule. It is the tumour extent which governs the level of division of the trachea.

147 **Suture materials:**
- A A suture of size 3/0 (BP) has a minimum suture diameter (MSD) of 0.2 mm
- B Nowadays, catgut is mostly synthetic
- C Absorbable sutures lose their tensile strength well before they finally dissolve
- D Synthetic absorbable sutures excite less inflammatory reaction than catgut
- E Silk is mostly obtained from proteinaceous thread spun by silkworm larvae

148 **Tree pollen allergy:**
- A Birch pollen is the most important cause of seasonal allergic rhinitis in Scandinavia
- B Pine tree pollen is an important cause of allergic rhinitis in Scotland
- C Tree pollens share most allergen loci
- D Tree pollen allergy is easily confirmed by RAST
- E Tree pollen allergy occurs before the start of the hay fever season

149 **The recurrent laryngeal nerve:**
- A The left nerve winds around the ligamentum arteriosum
- B Is motor to all the intrinsic laryngeal musculature
- C Is entirely motor
- D Is invariably intermingled with the terminal branches of the inferior thyroid artery
- E Gives branches to the cardiac plexus

150 **Tumours of the external ear:**
- A Ceruminomas may become malignant
- B Multiple osteomata in the external ear canal are associated with swimming
- C Squamous cell neoplasms of the external auditory canal are associated with a chronically discharging ear
- D Adenocarcinomas may occur following malignant transformation of a papilloma
- E Rodent ulcers do not occur in the external auditory meatus

151 **Infectious mononucleosis:**
- A Is caused by a virus
- B Is characterized by the presence of atypical monocytes on the blood film
- C Ampicillin is contraindicated
- D Spread is by the faeco-oral route
- E Abnormal liver function tests are common

147 A T The MSD of 10/0 is 0.02 mm and that of 0 is 0.35 mm.
    B F It is obtained from the intestine of sheep or cattle.
    C T
    D T And are absorbed more slowly in the tissue by a process of hydrolysis.
    E T

148 A T Ragweed is important in the USA and grass pollen in the UK.
    B F Pine trees cause allergic rhinitis in Japan but not elsewhere in the world.
    C F Tree pollens have different allergens for different species.
    D T The important trees for allergy are birch, plane, willow and hazel, and each one or a mixture must be tested. RAST gives accurate results.
    E T The tree pollen season is from early April until late May.

149 A T The right nerve does not enter the chest.
    B F Except cricothyroid.
    C F It is sensory to the laryngeal mucous membrane below the level of the vocal cords.
    D F This is an occasional finding. The nerve is more commonly found anterior to these branches and occasionally posterior.
    E T It also supplies part of the trachea and oesophagus.

150 A T Although most are benign, malignant transformation does occur.
    B T The occurrence of such osteomas is associated with the repeated entry of cold water into the meatus.
    C T In at least 75% of cases.
    D F Such a change would occur within an adenoma or ceruminoma.
    E F But they are not as common as the occurrence of squamous cell carcinomas.

151 A T The Epstein–Barr virus.
    B F Atypical lymphocytes.
    C T With ampicillin administration, a rash develops in over 95% and this is a diagnostic sign.
    D F It is by close contact, such as kissing.
    E T There may also be hepatosplenomegaly.

152   **Contraindications to the administration of corticosteroids include:**
A   Peptic ulceration
B   Iron deficiency anaemia
C   Severe hypertension
D   Otosclerosis
E   Pregnancy

153   **Perennial allergic rhinitis:**
A   Causes more complete nasal obstruction than does hay fever
B   Is more likely to be associated with asthma than is hay fever
C   Is usually not associated with grass pollen allergy
D   Has a major non-specific hyper-reactivity component
E   Is less severe in winter

154   **The pyriform fossa:**
A   Is bounded medially by the aryepiglottic fold
B   Is bounded laterally by the cricothyroid membrane
C   Constitutes a part of the laryngopharynx
D   Is closely related to branches of the internal laryngeal nerve
E   Malignant lesions are commoner in men

155   **Cerebellopontine angle tumours:**
A   Meningiomas are the commonest
B   Cholesteatoma in this region is thought to be 'secondary acquired'
C   Meningiomas are successfully treated with radiotherapy
D   The cerebellopontine angle is the most frequent intracranial site for the occurrence of meningiomas
E   Acoustic neuroma is a misnomer

156   **Tumours of the oral cavity:**
A   Lymphatic drainage of the tip of the tongue is primarily to the submental lymph glands
B   Lichen planus is premalignant
C   Adenocarcinoma is the commonest malignant lesion
D   Sarcomas would be treated with radiotherapy
E   A T_3 tongue tumour would imply spread across the midline

157   **Halothane:**
A   Causes hypertension
B   Can produce a postpartum haemorrhage
C   Causes liver damage
D   Is a respiratory tract irritant
E   Corrodes light metals

152   A T Others include diabetes mellitus, congestive cardiac failure, osteo-
        B F porosis and the immunocompromised patient.
        C T
        D F
        E T

153   A T Hay fever tends to produce only slight nasal obstruction.
        B T Asthma is frequently associated with perennial rhinitis.
        C F Grass pollen allergy is important in allergic perennial rhinitis.
        D T Perennial rhinitis is always associated with hyper-reactivity.
        E F The most important allergen of perennial rhinitis is the house dust
              mite and it is common in winter, especially early winter.

154   A T And also the quadrate membrane.
        B F Laterally are the thyroid cartilage and the thyrohyoid membrane.
        C T Along with the posterior pharyngeal wall and the postcricoid area.
        D T After they have pierced the thyrohyoid membrane.
        E T Postcricoid carcinoma, however, is commoner in women.

155   A F Acoustic neuromas are commoner.
        B F It is thought to be 'primary congenital'.
        C F Surgical excision is preferred since response to radiotherapy is poor.
        D F Only 7% occur here, yet they form 19% of all brain tumours.
        E T Vestibular schwannoma would be more apt.

156   A T The remaining anterior two thirds of the tongue drains directly to the
              deep cervical chain.
        B T Its erosive variety has a poorly defined relationship with the develop-
              ment of oral cancer.
        C F Squamous cell carcinoma is the commonest.
        D T
        E F Not necessarily. The 'T' classification of oral neoplasms is based on
              size only.

157   A F Its hypotensive effect can be used to reduce blood loss.
        B T It produces marked relaxation of the uterus.
        C T Especially after repeated administration. It should not, therefore, be
              administered to anyone who has received a previous halothane
              anaesthetic within a minimum of 4 weeks and, ideally, 6 months.
        D F It is non-irritant and induction is not unpleasant.
        E T In a moist atmosphere halothane corrodes (e.g. zinc, tin and
              aluminium), ruining any moving parts.

158 **Myringoplasty:**
- A   Is not a tympanoplasty
- B   Is a surgical repair of a tympanic membrane perforation
- C   Success is reduced in the presence of a poorly functioning eustachian tube
- D   The middle ear cavity is not entered when the 'onlay' technique is employed
- E   The presence of discharge in the middle ear cavity helps to secure the graft in position

159 **Cocaine:**
- A   Inhibits reuptake of endogenous catecholamines at the nerve terminal
- B   Has alpha- and beta-adrenoceptor agonist effects
- C   The topical vasoconstrictor effect is increased by the addition of adrenaline
- D   Causes local anaesthesia of the nasal vestibule
- E   Is toxic at topical doses in excess of 200 mg

160 **Caloric testing:**
- A   The patient lies on a couch with the head 30° above the horizontal
- B   Each irrigation should last for 40 s
- C   The time that is measured is from the end of irrigation until nystagmus is no longer detectable
- D   The fast component of the nystagmus beats towards the irrigated ear when using water at 30° C
- E   There should be at least a 5 min delay between each irrigation

161 **Teeth:**
- A   There are 20 deciduous teeth in total
- B   The first permanent tooth to erupt is a molar
- C   The inferior alveolar artery is a branch of the mandibular artery
- D   After bone, enamel is the next hardest animal substance in existence
- E   The lower molars each have 3 cusps

162 **Acute epiglottitis:**
- A   Only occurs in children
- B   Is usually caused by *Streptococcus pneumoniae*
- C   Has a peak age incidence between 18 months and 3 years
- D   Is characterized by a moderate fever
- E   Initial management consists of parenteral antibiotic therapy

163 **Myocardial infarction:**
- A   The pain is usually relieved by glyceryl trinitrate
- B   An anterior infarction shows ECG changes in leads II, III and AVF
- C   May be complicated by ventricular fibrillation
- D   Most deaths occur between 3 and 7 days
- E   S–T segment elevation on the ECG usually resolves within 4 weeks

158   A F A myringoplasty is a type I tympanoplasty (Wullstein classification).
      B T This is its definition.
      C T Best results occur when the tympanum is well aerated.
      D T It is the 'underlay' technique in which the middle ear is entered. The 'onlay' technique has been discredited due to cholesteatoma production.
      E F Otorrhoea is a contraindication for surgery and the best results are obtained in a dry ear.

159   A T Catecholamines are removed from the nerve terminal by reuptake and by 2 enzymes – catechol-O-methyltransferase and monoamine oxidase. Cocaine inhibits reuptake, making more catecholamine available at the nerve terminal, thus leading to vasoconstriction.
      B T
      C F Studies have shown that a maximal response is obtained by cocaine alone.
      D F Cocaine crosses mucous membranes but not skin.
      E T Cocaine is absorbed in toxic amounts when more than 3 mg/kg is applied to mucosal surfaces.

160   A T To bring the lateral semicircular canal into a vertical plane.
      B T
      C F The time is measured from the start of the irrigation.
      D F Remember 'COWS' – Cold Opposite, Warm Same.
      E T To enable the labyrinth to recover to its normal resting state.

161   A T There are five teeth in each half-jaw.
      B T At 6 years.
      C F It is a branch of the maxillary artery.
      D F It is the hardest.
      E F They each have two. The upper molars each have 3 cusps.

162   A F It also occurs in adults, although less frequently.
      B F The offending organism is invariably *Haemophilus influenzae* type B. In adults, however, streptococci and staphylococci have also been in implicated.
      C F It is 3–6 years.
      D F The fever is high.
      E F The airway should be secured primarily. Only then should the appropriate antibiotic therapy be commenced.

163   A F Unlike angina pectoris, myocardial infarction pain is not relieved by glyceryl trinitrate tablets or rest.
      B F Changes in these leads would indicate an inferior infarction. An anterior infarction would exhibit changes in leads I, II, AVL and V2–4.
      C T Or any other arrhythmia.
      D F Most deaths occur in the first hour following infarction.
      E T But Q and T wave changes resolve more slowly and may even remain permanently.

164 **Chronic non-suppurative otitis media:**
   A   May be a presenting feature of malignant disease
   B   Is associated with a sensorineural deafness
   C   Adenoidectomy may be a predisposing factor
   D   A second grommet insertion is seldom required
   E   May lead to cholesteatoma formation

165 **Malignant tonsil neoplasms:**
   A   Are more commonly squamous cell carcinomas
   B   Frequently present with metastases
   C   There is an increased incidence of a second tumour occurring
       within the respiratory tract
   D   Reticuloses present with ulceration
   E   Repair of a surgical defect is impractical

166 **Nasal polyposis is frequently associated with:**
   A   Asthma
   B   Chronic bronchitis
   C   Maxillary sinusitis
   D   Eczema
   E   Hay fever

167 **Ossiculoplasty:**
   A   A 'PORP' extends from the tympanic membrane to the footplate
       of the stapes
   B   A malleostapediopexy describes an interposition between the
       malleus handle and the head of the stapes
   C   A normally functioning eustachian tube is necessary for
       satisfactory restoration of hearing
   D   In the presence of a perforation of the tympanic membrane, an
       ossiculoplasty should be performed at the same time as the
       myringoplasty
   E   Sculptured ossicles give good long-term results

168 **The thyroid gland:**
   A   Is ensheathed by the deep investing layer of fascia
   B   Recurrent laryngeal nerve damage associated with
       thyroidectomy affects the left nerve 4 times more frequently
       than the right nerve
   C   Moves up and down during swallowing because embryologically
       the gland is derived from the foramen caecum of the tongue
   D   Colloid is a product of the follicular cells
   E   Can have a blood supply directly from the aortic arch

169 **Leucoplakia:**
   A   Is a white patch which cannot be scraped off
   B   Is premalignant
   C   May spontaneously regress
   D   May disappear with radiotherapy
   E   Should be kept under close observation

164   A   T   A nasopharyngeal neoplasm may cause a middle ear effusion because of eustachian tube obstruction.
      B   F   Conductive deafness is typical and is seldom greater than 40 dB.
      C   T   Over-zealous adenoidectomy may damage the eustachian cushion.
      D   F   A second grommet is required in up to 35% of cases.
      E   T   In cases of unrelieved or persistent middle ear effusions in which retractions may develop.

165   A   T   Constituting approximately 90%.
      B   T   Up to 75% present with lymph node metastases.
      C   T   Which are found either at the same time or at a later date in up to 20%.
      D   F   Ulceration is exceptional.
      E   F   A variety of flaps can be successfully employed.

166   A   T   70% of nasal polyposis sufferers have asthma.
      B   F
      C   T   60% of patients with nasal polyposis have infection of one or both maxillary antra as diagnosed by proof puncture.
      D   F
      E   F   Nasal polyposis is not an allergic condition.

167   A   F   This describes a 'TORP' – total ossicular replacement prosthesis – as opposed to a partial prosthesis which extends onto the head of the stapes.
      B   T
      C   T   Otherwise results are disappointing.
      D   F   Best results occur when the tympanic membrane is intact, although certain circumstances may allow relaxation of this rule.
      E   T   They usually become covered with mucous membrane and then become vascularized and viable.
      B   F   The incidence is equal.
      C   F   It is because the gland is invested with pretracheal fascia, thus the gland moves with the larynx on deglutition.
      D   T   The parafollicular or C cells produce thyrocalcitonin.
      E   T   The thyroidea ima artery may arise directly from the aortic arch in a few individuals and enters the lower part of the isthmus.

169   A   T   The white patch of candidiasis is easily removed.
      B   T   Although not all areas of leucoplakia become malignant.
      C   T   If a stimulus, such as smoking, is removed.
      D   F   Malignant transformation may follow radiotherapy.
      E   T   In order to note any malignant transformation at an early stage.

170 **Benign paroxysmal positional vertigo:**
    A   Is provoked by certain positions of the head
    B   May occur as a late sequel of acute otitis media
    C   Positional testing will show the nystagmus to beat towards the downmost ear
    D   Slowly worsens with time
    E   Is relieved by steroids

171 **Surgical diathermy:**
    A   In unipolar diathermy the current passes through the patient via an indifferent electrode directly to earth
    B   The diathermy electrodes become hot during use
    C   In bipolar diathermy the indifferent electrode is dispensed with
    D   The principal effects on the tissues are coagulation, fulguration and cutting
    E   Coagulation is used to seal blood vessels

172 **Chronic sensorineural deafness:**
    A   Presbyacusis occurs as a consequence of neuronal degeneration
    B   Presbyacusis is characterized by a hearing loss in the higher frequencies
    C   A quiet room is usually preferred to a noisy environment
    D   Is associated with hyperthyroidism
    E   Occurs in Paget's disease

173 **Functions of the liver include:**
    A   Platelet manufacture
    B   Hormone production
    C   Bile storage
    D   Manufacture of plasma proteins
    E   Urea formation

174 **Congenital deafness:**
    A   The time of maximal risk from rubella is the second trimester
    B   Rubella causes destruction of the organ of Corti
    C   Kernicterus typically causes a low tone deafness
    D   Rubella mostly affects hearing in the higher frequencies
    E   May be caused by syphilis

175 **Indications for tonsillectomy:**
    A   Psoriasis
    B   Glandular fever
    C   Glossopharyngeal neuralgia
    D   Recurrent pharyngitis
    E   Ludwig's angina

170   A   T   This is characteristic.
         B   T   It is the most common vestibular disturbance following closed head injury. It may occur spontaneously or following any insult to the ear.
         C   T   And may be accompanied by violent vertigo.
         D   F   The tendency is towards improvement.
         E   F   Relief is obtained by the avoidance of the offending position but provocation of the vertigo is the best treatment.

171   A   F   From the patient it passes back to the diathermy machine to the neutral pole of the generator and then to earth.
         B   F   It is only the tissues between the two electrodes that are heated.
         C   T   The two blades are separated by insulating material and together form an integral diathermy unit.
         D   T
         E   T   It is the simple application of heat and the consequent drying out of cells in the walls of the blood vessels, resulting in contraction.

172   A   T   But more commonly occurs from cochlear degeneration and recruitment would then be present.
         B   T   Especially those over 2 kHz.
         C   T   Patients with a conductive deafness prefer a noisy room; to those with a sensorineural deafness in a noisy room, however, the sounds are often unintelligible.
         D   F   It can occur in hypothyroidism.
         E   T   The otic capsule is included in up to 50% of cases.

173   A   F   Platelets are formed in the bone marrow.
         B   F   The liver produces no hormones.
         C   F   Bile is manufactured in the liver and stored in the gall bladder.
         D   T   Including those concerned with blood clotting.
         E   T   The urea is then excreted.

174   A   F   The risk of deafness is slight when rubella is acquired after the third month.
         B   T
         C   F   The cochlear nuclei are affected, resulting mainly in a high tone loss.
         D   F   The chief loss is usually in the middle frequencies.
         E   T   Either as a manifestation of secondary syphilis in the first 2 years of life or of tertiary syphilis, occurring between 8 and 20 years, or even later.

175   A   T   Relief is obtained in a proportion of cases.
         B   F   Only if later complicated by recurrent tonsillitis.
         C   T   Division of the nerve is possible via the tonsil fossa.
         D   F   Only if complicated by tonsillitis.
         E   F   The tonsils are not involved.

176 **The following exanthemata cause rhinitis:**
  A   Mumps
  B   Measles
  C   Chickenpox
  D   Rubella
  E   Smallpox

177 **The following are nasal muscles:**
  A   Procerus
  B   Levator labii superioris alaeque nasi
  C   Levator labii superioris
  D   Orbicularis oris
  E   Depressor septi

178 **The following structures pass between the internal and external carotid arteries:**
  A   Stylopharyngeus
  B   Glossopharyngeal nerve
  C   Posterior belly of digastric
  D   Vagus nerve
  E   Superior laryngeal nerve

179 **The organ of Corti:**
  A   Is supported by the basilar membrane
  B   The scala vestibuli is related to the under-surface of the basilar membrane
  C   There are more outer hair cells than inner hair cells
  D   The cilia of the hair cells are attached by their tips to the under-surface of Reissner's membrane
  E   The tunnel of Corti contains cortilymph

180 **Acute frontal sinusitis:**
  A   Typically pain is present in the evenings
  B   Supra-orbital pain from sinusitis is always due to frontal sinusitis
  C   Purulent secretions are usually seen within the middle meatus
  D   Oedema of the forehead is rare
  E   Does not cause headache

181 **Operative considerations in head and neck surgery:**
  A   The vertical limb of a Hayes–Martin type skin incision for a radical neck dissection should be 'S'-shaped
  B   Platysma should not be included in the skin flaps
  C   A Mcfee incision is suited for the patient who has received radiotherapy
  D   In continuity resection is not appropriate to the head and neck
  E   The skin incision should be marked with a pen as a preliminary

68 Answers

176 A F
     B T
     C T
     D T
     E T

177 A T The nasal muscles are procerus, nasalis, levator labii superioris
     B T alaeque nasi, depressor septi and the anterior and posterior dilator
     C F nares.
     D F
     E T

178 A T Other structures include the styloid process, styloglossus, the
     B T pharyngeal branch of the vagus and part of the parotid gland.
     C F
     D F
     E F

179 A T
     B F It is the scala tympani which is so related.
     C T About 4 times as many.
     D F They are attached to the tectorial membrane.
     E T It is chemically similar to perilymph.

180 A F Pain usually starts in the morning and subsides as the day progresses.
     B F It may also be caused by infection in the maxillary sinus.
     C F The frontonasal duct is usually occluded.
     D F
     E F Oedema over the forehead and headaches are common.

181 A T So that subsequent contraction will pull the incision to a straight line
            rather than a web.
     B F Platysma helps to give thickness and blood supply to the overlying
            skin.
     C T To prevent skin necrosis.
     D F Loss of continuity contravenes the principles of cancer surgery.
     E T During sewing up of the skin edges, marked distortion can occur.
            Tattooing helps to avoid this.

182 **Bell's palsy:**
  A   Is usually caused by a virus
  B   A partial paralysis is a good prognostic sign
  C   Lacrimation is usually absent on the affected side
  D   Is associated with a conductive deafness
  E   In most patients there is a neurotmesis

183 **The hypoglossal nerve:**
  A   Emerges as one nerve between the pyramid and the olive
  B   Leaves the skull through the jugular foramen
  C   Crosses the lingual artery above the greater cornu of the hyoid
  D   When injured, the tongue deviates towards the affected side during protrusion
  E   A palsy results in loss of taste to the anterior two thirds of the tongue on the affected side

184 **Intravenous barbiturates:**
  A   Thiopentone is long-acting
  B   Thiopentone is excreted by the kidneys
  C   May lead to gangrene of a limb
  D   Methohexitone is characterized by rapid effect and recovery
  E   Thiopentone is a powerful respiratory depressant

185 **The bony floor of the nose is formed by:**
  A   The palatal process of the palatine bone
  B   The horizontal process of the palatine bone
  C   The palatal process of the maxillary bone
  D   The palatal process of the ethmoid bone
  E   The horizontal process of the ethmoid bone

186 **Nasopharyngeal carcinoma:**
  A   Is more common than benign tumours of the nasopharynx
  B   Has a specific geographical distribution
  C   Deafness may be a presenting feature
  D   Lymphatic spread occurs more frequently than does haematogenous spread
  E   The muscles of mastication may be weak on the affected side

187 **Little's area (Kiesselbach's plexus) is an anastomosis of the following vessels:**
  A   Anterior ethmoidal
  B   Septal branch of superior labial
  C   Septal branch of greater palatine
  D   Septal branch of sphenopalatine
  E   Posterior ethmoidal

182   A   F   It is idiopathic by definition.
B   T   Recovery in this instance would be more favourable than if the original paralysis was complete.
C   F   It may be reduced but is seldom absent.
D   F   There is no known association.
E   F   80–85% develop a reversible neurapraxia.

183   A   F   It emerges as a linear series of 10–15 rootlets.
B   F   It has its own hypoglossal canal in the occipital bone.
C   T   After it has crossed the internal and external carotid arteries.
D   T   Due to the unopposed action of the contralateral muscles.
E   F   Taste sensation to this area is via the chorda tympani branch of the facial nerve.

184   A   F   It is ultra-short acting.
B   F   Not to any degree. Recovery from a dose depends on its destruction by metabolic processes.
C   T   If injected intra-arterially. The patient will complain of a sudden intense burning pain in the arm and hand.
D   T   It is thus very suitable for use in the outpatient and dental departments.
E   T

185   A   F   The anterior three quarters is formed by the palatal process of the
B   T   maxillary bone while the posterior quarter is formed by the
C   T   horizontal process of the palatine bone.
D   F
E   F

186   A   T   Much commoner. Juvenile angiofibroma is the only benign tumour of significance.
B   T   There is a high incidence in South China and Hong Kong.
C   T   Unilateral secretory otitis media in an adult should arouse one's suspicions.
D   T   A 'gland in the neck' is not an uncommon presentation.
E   T   The mandibular nerve at the foramen ovale becomes involved as the lesion expands.

187   A   T   Little's area is an anastomosis of the vessels mentioned except for the
B   T   posterior ethmoidal.
C   T
D   T
E   F

188 **The oesophagus:**
   A   Commences opposite the fourth cervical vertebra
   B   The cervical oesophagus receives its blood supply from oesophageal branches of the inferior thyroid artery
   C   The cervical oesophagus has the same neurovascular supply as the trachea
   D   The thoracic oesophagus is traversed by the right main bronchus
   E   The abdominal oesophagus is approximately 5 cm in length

189 **Tympanogram patterns:**
   A   Ossicular discontinuity exhibits an increased compliance
   B   Serous otitis media shows a normally-shaped graph but with a decreased compliance
   C   A tympanic membrane perforation exhibits a flat graph in the presence of a patent eustachian tube
   D   Otosclerosis offers the same pattern as that of a normal ear
   E   An occluded eustachian tube exhibits a flat graph

190 **Chronic suppurative otitis media:**
   A   The 'tubotympanic' type is not associated with complications
   B   Granulations occur more frequently in 'attico-antral' disease
   C   'Attico-antral' disease is more likely to be associated with a hypocellular mastoid
   D   The primary aim of treatment for 'attico-antral' disease is to restore hearing to normality
   E   Cholesteatoma does not occur in 'tubotympanic' disease

191 **Nasal allergy:**
   A   Is only occasionally associated with asthma
   B   Is associated with an increased risk of aspirin sensitivity
   C   Commonly leads to hypertrophy of the inferior turbinates
   D   An attack may be prevented by pretreatment with topical nasal steroid
   E   Is more common in patients who were not breast-fed as infants

192 **Hormones secreted by the pituitary gland include:**
   A   Oxytocin
   B   Melanotropin
   C   Thyrotrophin-releasing hormone
   D   Aldosterone
   E   Gastrin

193 **Stapedectomy:**
   A   May be complicated by total deafness
   B   Will improve a conductive deafness due to congenital stapedial fixation
   C   A 'safety hole' should be made in the footplate prior to division of the incudostapedial joint and the stapedial tendon
   D   Is usually contraindicated in the 'only hearing ear'
   E   Is the same as a stapedotomy

188 A F It is the sixth cervical vertebra.
  B T Its blood drains into the brachiocephalic veins.
  C T The nerve supply is from the recurrent laryngeal nerve.
  D F It is crossed by the left main bronchus.
  E F It is approximately 1.25 cm long.

189 A T As the tympanic membrane has an increased mobility.
  B F Typical findings are a negative middle ear pressure and a flat curve.
  C F It is not possible to obtain an airtight seal, thus recording is not possible.
  D F The graph is normally shaped but the compliance is reduced.
  E F The graph is normally shaped but it peaks at a negative pressure value.

190 A T It is the 'attico-antral' type that may develop complications.
  B T
  C T In 'tubotympanic' disease the mastoid is more likely to be well aerated.
  D F It is to render the ear safe and to prevent complications. Restoration of hearing is a secondary consideration.
  E F But it is uncommon.

191 A F There is a frequent association.
  B F Eosinophilic vasomotor rhinitis is associated with aspirin sensitivity but the latter is not an allergic phenomenon.
  C T Nasal obstruction is a frequent accompaniment of perennial allergic rhinitis.
  D T Pretreatment with topical steroids is effective at reducing the risk of an allergic reaction.
  E T Breast-fed infants seem to protect against allergy, perhaps by reducing the exposure to allergens, e.g. cow's milk.

192 A T Secreted by the posterior lobe.
  B T Secreted by the intermediate lobe.
  C F Secreted by the hypothalamus.
  D F Secreted by the adrenal.
  E F Secreted by the stomach and duodenum.

193 A T Even in experienced hands, a figure of 2% is quoted.
  B T But results are better for otosclerosis.
  C T Lest the footplate should mobilize and 'float'.
  D T A hearing aid is usually preferred.
  E F For a stapedotomy, the steps of a stapedectomy are more or less carried out in reverse order so that the prosthesis is in position before the stapes suprastructure is removed.

194 **Blastomycosis:**
    A   Usually starts in the lungs
    B   The most common extrapulmonary lesion is a verrucous ulcer with a serpiginous raised border affecting the skin
    C   Is caused by *Blastomyces dermatitidis*
    D   May be misdiagnosed as a carcinoma when occurring in the larynx
    E   Tends to invade the nose more frequently than histoplasmosis

195 **Tracheostomy teechnique:**
    A   A transverse incision is made at the level of the cricoid cartilage
    B   The thyroid isthmus should always be divided
    C   The neck should be extended as fully as possible
    D   The tracheostomy tube is secured in position while the neck is extended
    E   The first strap muscle to be visualized is sternothyroid

196 **The cavernous sinus:**
    A   Contains air
    B   Is a symmetrical structure
    C   The abducent nerve runs forwards towards the orbit medial to the internal carotid artery
    D   Drains by three emerging venous channels
    E   The maxillary is the most inferior of the nerves of those on the lateral wall

197 **The tympanic membrane:**
    A   Is composed of three layers
    B   Has a sensory nerve supply in part from the great auricular nerve
    C   Lies obliquely at 75° to the floor of the external auditory meatus
    D   The tympanic annulus is circumferential
    E   Its blood supply is from branches of the external carotid artery

198 **The ethmoidal arteries:**
    A   Pierce the lamina papyracea
    B   The foramen for the anterior ethmoidal artery lies 1 cm posterior to the maxillolacrimal suture
    C   The foramen for the posterior ethmoidal foramen is 1 cm posterior to the anterior ethmoidal foramen
    D   The posterior ethmoidal artery supplies the ethmoidal sinuses but not the nose
    E   Are branches of the optic artery

199 **Acute laryngotracheobronchitis:**
    A   Is best treated with antibiotics
    B   Exudate obstructs the tracheobronchial tree
    C   Laryngeal obstruction is usually rapid
    D   There is an associated cervical lymphadenopathy
    E   Occurs more frequently than acute epiglottitis

194   A   T The lung is the usual portal of entry.
      B   T
      C   T
      D   T Both the growth and the histopathologic features of the lesion resemble those of a well-differentiated carcinoma in the upper airway.
      E   F It occurs less frequently than histoplasmosis.

195   A   F It should be 2 cm below this.
      B   F It may be possible to displace it.
      C   T This facilitates surgery by making the trachea as superficial as possible.
      D   F It should be flexed prior to tying the tapes, otherwise they will slacken when neck flexion occurs.
      E   F It is sternohyoid.

196   A   F It contains venous blood.
      B   T And it lies alongside the body of the sphenoid bone.
      C   F It courses along its lateral aspect.
      D   T These are the superior and inferior petrosal sinuses, and a vein draining into the pterygoid plexus.
      E   T Followed superiorly by the ophthalmic, trochlear and oculomotor nerves.

197   A   T The pars tensa has an outer squamous epithelial layer, a middle fibrous layer and an inner layer of mucous membrane.
      B   F This nerve only supplies the pinna.
      C   F It lies at an angle of 55°.
      D   F It is deficient superiorly at the notch of Rivinus.
      E   T From the posterior auricular and maxillary arteries.

198   A   F The ethmoidal arteries pierce the fronto-ethmoid suture or, in some cases, the frontal bone itself.
      B   F The anterior ethmoidal foramen lies 14–22 mm posterior to the maxillofacial suture.
      C   T The posterior ethmoidal foramen lies 3–13 mm posterior to the anterior ethmoidal foramen.
      D   F It supplies ethmoidal air cells and the area of the superior turbinate.
      E   F They are branches of the ophthalmic artery derived from the internal carotid system.

199   A   F It has a viral aetiology.
      B   T And, along with oedema, causes stridor.
      C   F It is more usually slow and progressive.
      D   F This is unusual.
      E   T Much more frequently.

200 **Cimetidine:**
   A   Is an H_2 receptor antagonist
   B   Potentiates the effect of warfarin
   C   Relieves the symptoms of gastric carcinoma
   D   Is excreted by the kidney
   E   Is effective in the treatment of reflux oesophagitis

201 **Mastoiditis:**
   A   Acute mastoiditis occurs when the mucous membrane of the mastoid becomes inflamed
   B   Masked mastoiditis is said to occur when acute mastoiditis is associated with acute otitis externa
   C   Latent mastoiditis is associated with inadequate antibiotic therapy
   D   Chronic mastoiditis is associated with recurrent attacks of acute otitis media
   E   Acute mastoiditis usually occurs in the presence of a normal tympanic membrane

202 **Animal dander allergy:**
   A   Is due to allergy to animal hair
   B   Is due to allergy to animal skin scales
   C   Is due to allergy to a mite living on the skin of the animal
   D   Allergy to cat dander occurs in 20–30% of those suffering with allergic rhinitis
   E   Cat dander disappears from a house 3 months after removal of the animal

203 **The phrenic nerve:**
   A   Is a branch of the vagus nerve
   B   Passes downwards and almost vertically across the front of scalene anterior, over the prevertebral fascia
   C   Passes across the dome of the pleura behind the subclavian vein
   D   Gives off branches in the neck
   E   Contains motor and sensory nerve fibres

204 **Neck glands associated with an 'occult' primary:**
   A   The most frequent primary site is the base of the tongue
   B   The primary site is always in the head and neck region
   C   The primary site eventually becomes evident in most cases
   D   Should be excised as a first step
   E   Long-term follow-up is necessary

205 **Viral infections of the upper respiratory tract:**
   A   Rhinoviruses are the main cause of the common cold
   B   Respiratory syncitial virus is a frequent cause of bronchiolitis in infants less than 1 year of age
   C   Echoviruses cause acute laryngotracheobronchitis
   D   Pharyngitis and conjunctivitis are the main respiratory tract symptoms of the rhinovirus
   E   Coronaviruses cause up to 10% of 'colds' in the community

200 A T Leading to a reduction of gastric acid secretion by about 80%.
     B T And certain beta-blockers.
     C T Thus it should not be prescribed until this diagnosis has been excluded.
     D T Thus caution should be applied in patients with renal disorders.
     E T Although the response rate is less than for peptic ulceration.

201 A F It occurs when there is coalescence of air cells and invariably leads to the formation of an empyema. It cannot occur in the absence of air cells.
     B F It is invariably due to failed antibiotic therapy for acute otitis media and is associated with persistent otorrhoea.
     C T After apparent recovery from acute suppurative otitis media, the latter recurs several weeks later and may then present as mastoiditis.
     D F It is a complication of chronic suppurative otitis media and is a slow penetration of acellular bone by granulation tissue, accompanied by hyperaemic decalcification.
     E F Abnormality of the tympanic membrane is invariably present.

202 A F Animal dander allergy is due to a mite living on the skin scales of the
     B F animal. It has even been suggested that the actual allergen is a mite
     C T living on the mite!
     D T Cat dander allergy is the commonest and most troublesome animal dander allergy.
     E F It takes at least 1 year for the allergen to disappear in a house.

203 A F It is derived from the third, fourth and fifth cervical nerves.
     B F It lies behind the prevertebral fascia.
     C T And in front of the subclavian artery.
     D F There are no branches in the neck.
     E T It is motor to the diaphragm and sensory to related areas of parietal pleura, pericardium and peritoneum.

204 A F It is the nasopharynx.
     B F It may rarely be the bronchus, oesophagus, breast or stomach.
     C T It is not found in one third of patients.
     D F A thorough examination of the upper aerodigestive tract should be undertaken primarily, including examination under general anaesthesia if necessary.
     E T The primary site may become manifest many years later.

205 A T
     B T It may also cause pneumonia.
     C F This is usually caused by parainfluenza viruses.
     D F They are more typical of adenoviruses.
     E T Although there is difficulty in isolating them.

206 **Olfactory cognition:**
    A   Odour associations tend to linger in the memory much longer than associations from the other senses
    B   Children are born with an innate dislike of unpleasant odours
    C   Children as young as 6 days of age are able to recognize their mother by smell
    D   Adaptation to odours occurs in about 15 min
    E   In women the sense of smell is more acute at ovulation

207 **Tumours of the middle ear and mastoid:**
    A   There is no known predisposing factor
    B   Adenocarcinoma is the commonest form of primary tumour
    C   Bleeding is an uncommon feature
    D   May have the appearance of an innocent-looking polyp
    E   Rhabdomyosarcoma is a slowly-growing tumour in this area

208 **The posterior cervical triangle:**
    A   Is bounded posteriorly by the anterior border of trapezius
    B   Is divided into a lower supraclavicular triangle and an upper carotid triangle by the inferior belly of omohyoid
    C   The phrenic nerve courses over levator scapulae
    D   Its apical lymph nodes tend to enlarge during rubella
    E   Its roof is formed by the deep investing layer of cervical fascia

209 **Blood:**
    A   Platelets have a half-life of about 21 days
    B   The average total circulatory blood volume is 3000 ml
    C   55% of the total circulating blood volume is plasma
    D   Megakaryocytes are platelet precursors
    E   Chemotaxis is the process whereby plasma factors act on bacteria to make them 'tasty' to the phagocytes

210 **Glomus tumours:**
    A   The most characteristic symptom of a glomus tympanicum is pulsatile tinnitus
    B   Glomus tympanicum tumours are usually associated with a perforation of the tympanic membrane
    C   A retrograde jugular venogram is an essential investigation
    D   Should be embolized prior to surgical resection
    E   May be excised surgically

211 **Rhinoscleroma:**
    A   Is caused by *Klebsiella rhinoscleromatis*
    B   Is endemic in Scandinavia
    C   Tends not to invade the larynx
    D   Produces a granulomatous mass in the nose
    E   Tends not to invade the external nose

206 A T Associations of odour may linger in the memory for a lifetime.
    B F This does not occur until about the age of 4 years.
    C T
    D F It occurs in 1–5 min.
    E T Olfactory acuity is most acute at ovulation and least acute at menstruation.

207 A F In the majority there is a history of chronic otorrhoea.
    B F Squamous cell carcinoma is more common, despite the low prevalence of squamous epithelium.
    C F Pain and bleeding are common features.
    D T Hence all polypi in the middle ear should be examined histologically.
    E F It is very aggressive, usually occurring in children and young adults.

208 A T
    B F Above omohyoid is the occipital triangle.
    C F It overlies scalene anterior.
    D T Or with scalp infections.
    E T It is also covered by skin, superficial fascia and platysma.

209 A F It is 4 days.
    B F It is 5600 ml in a 70 kg man.
    C T
    D T
    E F This is opsonization. Chemotaxis is the process whereby neutrophils are attracted to an infected area.

210 A T Followed by deafness, which is usually conductive.
    B F They are usually seen behind an intact tympanic membrane.
    C F Angiography will delineate the tumour and its blood supply. Its venous phase can assess the jugular bulb.
    D T This reduces the vascularity and thus facilitates surgical excision.
    E T Especially when employing skull-base surgical techniques, as developed by Fisch.

211 A T
    B F The disease is endemic in Western USA, Central America and Eastern Europe.
    C F 80% of subjects have laryngeal involvement.
    D T
    E F The lesion tends to be anterior and invades the lower external nose, causing severe disfigurement.

212 **Diabetes mellitus:**
A   Affects 1% of the population
B   'Juvenile onset' patients are usually insulin-dependent
C   Occurs in acromegaly
D   Polyuria is caused by an osmotic diuresis
E   Affected patients should be last on an operating list

213 **The parathyroid glands:**
A   Are usually four in number
B   Oxyphil cells secrete parathormone
C   Lie anterior to the thyroid gland
D   Have a nerve supply which is solely sympathetic
E   Parathormone secretion is related to the concentration of calcium ions in the blood supplying the glands

214 **Acute tonsillitis:**
A   Is associated with a leucocytosis
B   Associated otalgia is always referred pain
C   An elevated anti-streptolysin titre would indicate infection of a bacterial rather than a viral nature
D   Can occur following tonsillectomy
E   The most frequent lymph glands involved are those in the jugulodigastric region

215 **Tracheostomy:**
A   Humidification is essential in the immediate postoperative period
B   The patient may be artificially ventilated via a silver tracheostomy tube
C   The first tracheal ring may be excised
D   Pneumothorax is a complication
E   A Bjork flap is based superiorly

216 **Traumatic rupture of the tympanic membrane:**
A   May be caused by liquids
B   May be caused by air
C   May be associated with a sensorineural deafness
D   Spontaneous healing is usual
E   Blood in the external auditory canal which occludes the view of the tympanic membrane should be removed

217 **The maxillary sinus:**
A   Has a volume of approximately 5 ml
B   Has accessory ostia in 5% of individuals
C   Has a floor 1.5 cm below that of the nose
D   Has its largest dimension (anteroposterior) of 3.5 cm
E   Is bounded on all sides by the maxilla

212   A   T   At least.
    B   T   'Maturity onset' patients are usually controlled on diet alone or using oral hypoglycaemic agents.
    C   T   And also in Cushing's syndrome, phaeochromocytoma and glucagon-secreting tumours.
    D   T   As a result of the hyperglycaemia. Polydipsia follows.
    E   F   They should be first so that there is minimal fasting.

213   A   T
    B   F   Their function is unknown. Parathormone is secreted by the chief cells.
    C   F   They are situated posteriorly.
    D   T   It is probably vasomotor rather than secretomotor.
    E   T

214   A   T   Usually a polymorphonuclear leucocytosis.
    B   F   It may be due to an associated acute otitis media.
    C   T   This would indicate a streptococcal infection.
    D   T   Either due to lingual tonsillitis or inflammation in tonsil remnants.
    E   T   Lymphatic drainage is primarily to this area.

215   A   T   Otherwise crusting of secretions occurs, with subsequent tracheal obstruction.
    B   F   Silver tubes are not cuffed.
    C   F   Laryngotracheal stenosis will inevitably occur.
    D   T   It is important to remain close to the midline as the pleura rise in the neck.
    E   F   It is based inferiorly, but its use is not advised.

216   A   T   Frequently seen with too vigorous ear syringing.
    B   T   As in blast waves from explosions, 'slapping' the ear and in baro-trauma.
    C   T   In severe cases, such as a skull fracture, both the inner ear and the middle ear may be involved. There may be a temporary sensorineural deafness following 'blast' and 'slapping' injuries associated with a tympanic membrane perforation.
    D   T   As long as the perforation is not too large and there is no super-added infection.
    E   F   Blood acts as a good scaffolding for spontaneous healing to occur.

217   A   F   Its volume is 15 ml.
    B   F   In 25–30% of individuals there are accessory ostia, usually situated inferior to the uncinate process.
    C   F   Its floor is 4–5 mm inferior to the floor of the nose, on average, but may be as much as 1.25 cm.
    D   T   Its dimensions are 3.5 cm anteroposterior, 2.5 cm transverse and 3.3 cm high.
    E   F   All except a part of the medial wall, which is formed by the ethmoid.

218 **Rhinomanometry:**
    A   Involves measuring the nasal pressure gradient and the airflow rate simultaneously
    B   Is quick and easy to perform
    C   Can be used in low dose allergen testing challenge
    D   Is used as a routine in many major UK centres
    E   Is mainly used in rhinological research

219 **Syphilis:**
    A   *Treponema pallidum* is Gram-positive
    B   A primary chancre develops at the site of entry in the first week
    C   Secondary syphilis is characterized by a dull red macular or maculopapular rash
    D   A gumma is infectious
    E   There is no curative treatment

220 **Cranial autonomic ganglia:**
    A   The sympathetic roots are preganglionic
    B   The otic ganglion has a motor root supplying the tensor palati muscle
    C   The sensory root of the ciliary ganglion is a branch of the nasociliary nerve
    D   Postganglionic parasympathetic fibres of the submandibular ganglion are secretomotor to the sublingual gland
    E   Sympathetic fibres of the pterygopalatine ganglion supply the mucous glands of the nose

221 **Radical neck dissection:**
    A   Is the same operation as a block neck dissection
    B   The prevertebral fascia is removed
    C   Dissection commences in the supraclavicular triangle
    D   The blood supply to the levator scapulae enters the muscle anteriorly
    E   The lower end of the internal jugular vein is divided after it has been exposed by retracting the sternomastoid muscle

222 **The eustachian tube:**
    A   Its bony portion is twice as long as its cartilaginous segment
    B   Its nasopharyngeal ostium is supplied by the nervus spinosus branch of the mandibular nerve
    C   The internal carotid artery is medial to the bony portion
    D   Closes by the contraction of the levator palati
    E   Congenital absence is associated with first arch syndromes

218 A T
 B F If performed in the correct manner, a full and complete measurement on one patient will take up to 45 min.
 C T Very low doses of aqueous allergen can be introduced into the nose without causing the danger and discomfort of a high dose challenge. Small increases in nasal resistance can then be measured.
 D F Rhinomanometry is only occasionally performed routinely in the UK.
 E T

219 A F It cannot be Gram stained.
 B F It appears after an incubation period of 9–90 days.
 C T Other features include general malaise, condylomata lata, and 'snail track' ulcers on the palate or in the pharynx.
 D F It is a syphilitic hypersensitivity reaction and is the characteristic lesion of tertiary syphilis.
 E F Penicillin is curative.

220 A F They are postganglionic but the parasympathetic roots synapse in the ganglion.
 B T This root is a branch of the nerve to the medial pterygoid muscle. It also supplies tensor tympani.
 C T The cell bodies are in the trigeminal ganglion.
 D T
 E F These are supplied by the parasympathetic fibres. The sympathetic fibres are vasoconstrictor to the mucous membrane of the nose, nasopharynx, sinuses and palate.

221 A F A block dissection is removal of the primary tumour in continuity with an enlarged mass of nodes. It is short for 'en bloc'.
 B F If this layer is not breached the cervical nerve roots cannot be damaged.
 C T Followed by the occipital triangle.
 D T Thus the muscle can be swung forwards to protect the internal carotid artery.
 E F Sternomastoid is divided.

222 A F The bony portion is 12 mm in length and its cartilaginous portion is 24 mm long.
 B F It is supplied by the pharyngeal branch of the sphenopalatine ganglion. The nervus spinosus supplies its cartilaginous part and the tympanic plexus (glossopharyngeal nerve) supplies the bony part.
 C T
 D F This helps to open the tube along with tensor palati. In the resting phase the tube closes passively.
 E T Especially in the Treacher–Collins syndrome.

223 **Taste:**
- A   Taste buds disappear following denervation
- B   Taste buds are located in the mucosa of the epiglottis
- C   Bitter substances are tasted towards the back end of the anterior two thirds of the tongue
- D   Drugs may reduce taste sensation
- E   Acids taste bitter

224 **Herpes viruses:**
- A   The Epstein–Barr virus is a herpes virus
- B   All have the property of remaining latent
- C   Cause Creutzfeld-Jakob disease
- D   May cause deafness
- E   Cause molluscum contagiosum

225 **The stomach:**
- A   The greater curvature receives its blood supply from the gastric arteries
- B   Is lined with squamous stratified epithelium
- C   Its parasympathetic fibres are vasomotor and are inhibitory to gut muscle
- D   The pylorus is that part which projects upwards above the level of the cardiac orifice
- E   Has outer longitudinal and inner circular muscle coats

226 **Acute suppurative otitis media:**
- A   Is a complication of acute tonsillitis
- B   Myringotomy should be performed in the presence of a bulging tympanic membrane
- C   When complicated by a facial nerve paralysis, surgery is indicated
- D   Is usually associated with a conductive deafness
- E   Acute necrotizing otitis media may follow scarlet fever

227 **Important occupational allergens are:**
- A   Penicillin
- B   Trimellitic anhydride
- C   Formaldehyde
- D   Soft wood sawdust
- E   Platinum salts

228 **Antihypertensive therapy:**
- A   Atenolol is cardioselective
- B   Non-selective beta-blockers should not be prescribed to insulin-dependent diabetics
- C   Beta-blockers generally increase alertness and concentration
- D   Thiazide diuretics cause hypokalaemia
- E   Methyldopa causes postural hypotension

223 A T After they have degenerated.
    B T They also occur in the palate, oro- and hypopharynx, and tongue.
    C T Sour along the edges, sweet at the tip and salty anteriorly on the dorsum.
    D T Such as captopril and penicillamine, due to the presence of sulfhydryl groups.
    E F They taste sour. Sourness is generally proportionate to the hydrogen ion concentration.

224 A T As are the herpes simplex, varicella zoster and cytomegaloviruses.
    B T In a potentially viable form. They may persist throughout life.
    C F This is caused by a slow virus.
    D T Either from congenital cytomegalovirus infection or associated with the herpes zoster infection of the Ramsay Hunt syndrome.
    E F This is caused by a poxivirus.

225 A F Its blood supply is from the gastroepiploic arteries.
    B F It is lined with columnar epithelium.
    C F This describes the action of its sympathetic fibres. Its parasympathetic fibres are motor to the gut and secretomotor to the glands.
    D F This is the fundus.
    E T These invest the stomach and are reinforced by an incomplete, innermost, oblique muscle coat.

226 A T Recurrent attacks of acute suppurative otitis media associated with recurrent tonsillitis is an indication for tonsillectomy.
    B T There would be less long-term risk to the hearing and less tissue necrosis, but this procedure is, in fact, rarely performed.
    C F The palsy almost always recovers following therapy with parenteral antibiotics.
    D T Confirmed by tuning fork tests and audiometry.
    E T Or other exanthemata, and is invariably caused by a β-haemolytic streptococcus.

227 A T Penicillin is a hazard both to hospital workers and to those working in the pharmaceutical industry.
    B T Trimellitic anhydride is widely used in the manufacture of epoxy resins, paints and plastics. Its fumes produce both rhinitis and asthma.
    C F Formaldehyde is an irritant, not an allergen.
    D F Soft wood sawdust is not a hazard. Asthma is not uncommon in those working with hardwoods and the dust of the Western red cedar is particularly notorious.
    E T Complex platinum salts probably give rise to true allergic reactions and positive skin tests to these salts are common.

228 A T Thus bronchospasm is not usually a problem.
    B T As the symptoms of hypoglycaemia may be lost.
    C F They cause fatigue and weakness.
    D T And may precipitate cardiac arrhythmias, especially in patients concurrently taking digoxin.
    E T Especially in the elderly.

229 **The diaphragm:**
- A   Is supplied entirely by the phrenic nerve
- B   The oesophageal hiatus lies opposite the twelfth thoracic vertebra
- C   The oesophageal hiatus transmits the vagal nerve trunks
- D   The oesophageal hiatus is situated within the central tendon
- E   It plays its major role during expiration

230 **Ringertz tumours (inverting nasal papilloma):**
- A   Constitute approximately 10% of all nose and sinus neoplasms
- B   Do not erode bone
- C   Cause a sanguinous nasal discharge as the main symptom
- D   Are radiosensitive
- E   Exhibit epithelial inversion into the surrounding stroma when examined histologically

231 **Masking:**
- A   Is applied to the ear being tested
- B   Is mandatory for all bone conduction threshold tests
- C   Should be used whenever there is a loss of 50 dB or more at any frequency for air-conducted sounds
- D   Wide-band noise is the most efficient for masking pure tone stimuli
- E   'Overmasking' occurs when the masking noise leaks around the head to the cochlea of the test ear

232 **Acute laryngitis:**
- A   Is always initiated by an upper respiratory infection
- B   May require a tracheostomy
- C   Can be complicated by acute perichondritis of the laryngeal cartilages
- D   Usually resolves rapidly without the use of antibiotics
- E   Hoarseness is the commonest feature

233 **Respiration:**
- A   The tidal volume is the amount of air moving into the lungs during inspiration plus the amount moving out during expiration, during quiet respiration
- B   Diaphragmatic movement accounts for most of the change in intrathoracic volume during quiet inspiration
- C   Carbon dioxide is more soluble in blood than is oxygen
- D   Baroreceptors monitor the effects of variations in blood chemistry during ventilation
- E   Central chemoreceptors are situated in the pons

234 **The following disorders reduce the sense of smell:**
- A   Bell's palsy
- B   Chronic renal failure
- C   Hepatic cirrhosis
- D   Adrenal insufficiency
- E   Sjögren's syndrome

229   A   F   The lower intercostal nerves are sensory to its peripheral part.
      B   F   It lies opposite the tenth thoracic vertebra.
      C   T   Along with the oesophageal branches of the left gastric artery.
      D   F   This is the site of the caval opening. The oesophageal opening is surrounded by the crura (striated muscle).
      E   F   Its major role is during inspiration.

230   A   F   Ringertz tumours account for only 2% of tumours of the nose and sinuses.
      B   F   The tumour mass may cause pressure erosion of the surrounding bone.
      C   F   The lesion presents with nasal obstruction and appears as a firm red or grey mass.
      D   F   It is neither radiosensitive nor radiocurable and local excision is the first line of treatment.
      E   T

231   A   F   It is applied to the non-test ear.
      B   T   Since bone-conducted sound stimulates each cochlea with equal intensity.
      C   T   Air-conducted sound above this pressure level provokes skull vibration, i.e. it is attenuated across the head by 50 dB.
      D   F   The most efficient is white noise filtered to a narrow band, which is centred on the test frequency.
      E   T

232   A   F   Other causes include irritation (smoke and fumes) and vocal abuse.
      B   T   This is an important consideration in children.
      C   T   This is usually associated with a bacterial aetiology.
      D   T   Local treatments are usually adequate.
      E   T   It is the main presenting symptom.

233   A   F   It is one or the other, not both. Its average volume is 500 ml.
      B   T   About 75%.
      C   T   20 times more.
      D   F   This action is performed by the chemoreceptors.
      E   F   These receptor cells lie in the medulla in the floor of the fourth ventricle

234   A   F   Taste, not smell, is affected.
      B   T
      C   T
      D   F   Adrenal insufficiency tends to cause an increase in the ability to detect odours.
      E   T

235 **Support of the nasal tip is achieved by:**
A The shape and size of the alar cartilages
B The medial crural footplate attached to the caudal septum
C The attachment of the upper lateral cartilages to the alar cartilages
D The cartilaginous nasal septum
E The nasal spine

236 **The first rib:**
A Receives the attachment of scalene posterior
B Scalene anterior is attached to the scalene tubercle
C The subclavian groove is occupied by the subclavian artery
D The groove for the subclavian vein is anterior to the scalene tubercle
E Gives sole origin to serratus anterior

237 **Congenital abnormalities of the external ear:**
A The primary defect in the 'bat ear' is the absence of the concha
B Anotia is usually part of a second arch syndrome
C A preauricular fistula is usually caused by defective closure of the first branchial cleft
D Surgery is indicated in cases of bilateral meatal atresia in the presence of good bilateral cochlear function
E Occur in Down's syndrome

238 **Osteogenic sarcoma of the jaws:**
A Forms 7% of all cases of osteogenic sarcoma
B Has a predilection for the maxilla
C Tends to be painless
D Is controlled by radiotherapy
E Tends to metastasize to the lungs

239 **Causes of acute (sudden) sensorineural deafness include:**
A Acoustic neuroma
B Presbyacusis
C Infectious mononucleosis
D Acute secretory otitis media
E Otic barotrauma

240 **Hay fever:**
A Has doubled in incidence over the past 10 years
B Is more likely to occur in patients born during the hay fever season
C Is more difficult to treat once symptoms have been present for a week
D More severe cases may be treated with systemic steroids
E Tends to lessen with increasing age

88   *Answers*

235 A T The support of the nasal tip is achieved by structures of both major
     B T and minor importance. A, B and C are of major importance. In
     C T addition to the nasal spine, other structures of minor importance
     D F include interdomal soft tissue, the cartilaginous dorsum, the soft
     E T tissue–sesamoid complex attaching the lateral crus to the piriform
             wall, the alar cartilage attachment to the skin and soft tissue, and the
             membranous nasal septum.

236 A F This muscle is attached to the second rib.
     B T And also to an adjacent area on its upper surface.
     C F The subclavian groove lodges the lower trunk of the brachial plexus.
             The subclavian artery touches only the outer border of the first rib.
     D T
     E F Its muscular digitations arise from the outer surfaces and superior
             borders of the upper 8–10 ribs.

237 A F The antihelix is absent and a new antihelix should be reconstructed
             for good long-term results.
     B F Along with other abnormalities it usually forms part of a first arch
             syndrome.
     C T In 90% of cases the fistula opens close to the anterior border of the
             ascending helical limb.
     D T A unilateral atresia with a contralateral normal ear would certainly
             not require early surgery, if any.
     E T The pinna tends to be small and rounded in contour, with a poorly
             developed lobule.

238 A T
     B F It is more common in the mandible than in the maxilla.
     C F Growth is rapid and often painful. The tumour causes facial swelling
             and loosening of teeth.
     D F Surgical resection, with perhaps adjuvant chemotherapy, offers the
             best chance of cure.
     E T

239 A T In up to 10% of cases.
     B F Deafness is slow and progressive.
     C T Occurring as a part of the systemic illness.
     D F The deafness, although of acute onset, is conductive.
     E T If there is an associated rupture of the oval window or round window
             membrane.

240 A T Its incidence is rising but the reason is unclear.
     B T Early exposure to allergen when IgA is low offers poor defence for
             children born during the hay fever season.
     C T When inflammation has been present for some time it takes longer
             to control symptoms.
     D T Methylprednisolone depot injection or low dose prednisolone orally
             are effective in refractory cases and may be especially useful in specific
             circumstances, such as prior to examinations, but these measures
             should be avoided if possible.
     E T

241 **Drugs used in neurological disease:**
A   Levodopa may reverse the underlying disease process of Parkinsonism
B   Phenytoin causes nystagmus
C   Carbamazepine is effective in controlling temporal lobe epilepsy
D   Serotonin receptor antagonists are effective against an acute attack of migraine
E   Phenobarbitone causes nasal obstruction

242 **The styloid process:**
A   Gives origin to three muscles
B   The stylohyoid ligament extends to the lesser cornu of the hyoid
C   Is deep to the facial nerve
D   Averages 5 cm in length
E   Stylopharyngeus arises from the medial aspect of its base

243 **Postoperative care following head and neck surgery:**
A   Laryngectomy patients should be tube-fed for a minimum of 3 weeks
B   Following a laryngectomy-associated hemithyroidectomy, the serum calcium should be checked the following morning
C   Following a laryngectomy-associated hemithyroidectomy, the serum thyroxine should be checked the following morning
D   For cancer surgery, follow-up should be at least monthly for the first year
E   Following a laryngectomy all suction drains should be removed within 72 h of surgery

244 **Otogenic extradural abscess:**
A   May be asymptomatic
B   Is the most frequent otogenic intracranial complication
C   The usual cause is a retrograde septic thrombophlebitis
D   Only occurs in the middle cranial fossa
E   May give rise to Gradenigo's syndrome

245 **Squamous cell carcinoma of the sinuses:**
A   Tends to present early when occurring in the maxillary antrum
B   Tends to present early when occurring in the ethmoidal sinuses
C   Has a worse prognosis when occurring high within the ethmoids or maxillary antrum
D   Cervical lymph node metastases are common
E   Maxillary antral carcinoma is more frequently diagnosed once it has extended beyond the confines of the sinus

241 A F The efficacy of levodopa falls off with long-term treatment.
     B T At high plasma levels.
     C T It is also effective when used to treat trigeminal neuralgia.
     D F They are an effective prophylactic treatment. Symptomatic treatment is used for the acute attack.
     E F But it does cause vertigo, ataxia and sedation.

242 A T Stylohyoid, stylopharyngeus and styloglossus.
     B T Thus 'suspending' the hyoid from the skull.
     C T As the nerve passes from the stylomastoid foramen to the parotid gland.
     D F It is 2.5 cm in length.
     E T

243 A F About 7–10 days is sufficient in uncomplicated cases.
     B T Hypocalcaemia declares itself early.
     C F Hypothyroidism does not develop for at least a week post-operatively.
     D T Culminating in annual visits after 5 years.
     E F Drains should be removed when they no longer drain fluids.

244 A T It may be discovered by chance during a mastoidectomy.
     B T
     C F Bone separating the middle ear and mastoid from the intracranial space is most commonly destroyed by hyperaemic decalcification or by cholesteatomatous erosion.
     D F The posterior fossa may also be affected.
     E T Collections of pus may overlie the petrous apex.

245 A F Late presentation occurs more frequently.
     B T There is not as large a cavity for the tumour to fill before it breaks out.
     C T By the use of hypothetical lines dividing the ethmoids and antrum into supra-, meso- and infrastructure, tumours occurring in the suprastructure have a worse prognosis.
     D F Lymph node metastases are uncommon.
     E T Generally, symptoms occur only when the neoplasm has spread outside the bony walls of the sinus.

246 **Systemic lupus erythematosus:**
   A   Is commoner in men
   B   Is a cause of nasal septal ulceration
   C   Tends not to cause nasal septal perforations
   D   25% of patients will demonstrate a false-positive result when tested serologically for syphilis
   E   Gives a characteristic nasofacial rash which is triggered by sunlight

247 **The accessory nerve:**
   A   Overlies levator scapulae as it crosses the posterior triangle
   B   Its spinal root supplies the motor fibres to sternomastoid
   C   Its cranial root supplies motor fibres to tensor veli palatini
   D   Passes medial to the posterior belly of digastric
   E   Is proprioceptive to sternomastoid

248 **The Shah aural ventilation tube:**
   A   Has the same lumen diameter as the Shepard aural tube
   B   Inner and outer flanges are identical
   C   Its insertion requires a larger myringotomy incision than does that for the Shepard tube
   D   For ease of introduction, the outer flange should, ideally, be grasped
   E   Is made of silicone

249 **The parapharyngeal space:**
   A   Extends from the base of the skull to the clavicle
   B   Is situated between the nasopharynx and the inner surface of the angle and ascending ramus of the mandible
   C   Is continuous with the retropharyngeal space
   D   The carotid sheath and vessels lie in its prestyloid compartment
   E   The medial wall of the prestyloid compartment is formed by the buccopharyngeal fascia covering tensor palati and the superior constrictor

250 **Grass pollen allergy:**
   A   Occurs in up to 20% of the population
   B   Grass pollens share most allergen loci
   C   Moderately severe hay fever is best controlled with topical nasal steroids
   D   Hay fever is well controlled with nasal decongestants
   E   Hay fever is an important cause of time lost from school

246   A   F   It occurs in both sexes of all ages.
      B   T
      C   F   Nasal dryness and septal ulceration leading to septal perforation
              tend to occur.
      D   T
      E   T   The rash, occurring in approximately 50% of subjects, is red and
              crusty.

247   A   T
      B   T   And also to trapezius.
      C   F   But it does supply the other muscles of the soft palate.
      D   T   It also passes medial to the styloid process and stylohyoid.
      E   F   The second and third cervical nerves carry the proprioceptive fibres.

248   A   T   1.1 mm.
      B   F   The inner flange is longer and larger.
      C   F   Because the inner flange is tapered a smaller incision is required.
      D   F   The short process of the inner surface should be grasped.
      E   F   It is composed of teflon.

249   A   F   It extends inferiorly only to the level of the hyoid bone.
      B   T
      C   T
      D   F   They lie in the retrostyloid compartment, along with the last four
              cranial nerves, cervical sympathetic nerves and lymph nodes.
      E   T   And its floor is formed by the fascia investing the submandibular
              gland.

250   A   T   Grass pollen allergy is the most common allergic disease and must
              be considered a variant of normal.
      B   T   There are three major grass pollen loci on a grass pollen grain and
              these are shared by all the species of grass.
      C   T   Topical nasal steroids have been shown to provide superior control
              for hay fever than antihistamines. The latter block histamine, whereas
              topical nasal steroids block most of the other mediators, directly or
              indirectly.
      D   F   Nasal decongestants do not reduce the amount of inflammatory
              mediators and play little part in the management of hay fever.
      E   T   Hay fever is, indeed, an important cause of school absence and poor
              examination performance.

251 **Lymph:**
- A Lymphocytes enter the circulation principally through the lymphatics
- B Is tissue fluid that enters the lymphatic vessels
- C Does not clot
- D Water-soluble fats are absorbed from the intestine into the lymphatics
- E Lymph in the thoracic duct after a meal is milky

252 **The Wullstein tympanoplasty classification:**
- A A myringoplasty is a 'type 1'
- B In a 'type 4', the round window is shielded by a fascia graft but the entire stapes is exposed and mobile
- C A 'type 5' consists of fenestration of the lateral semicircular canal
- D In a 'type 2', a tympanomeatal flap or a fascial graft is placed upon the head of the stapes
- E In a 'type 2', sound is conducted through a deformed – but functioning – ossicular chain

253 **The bony lateral nasal wall is formed at least in part by:**
- A The nasal surface of the maxilla
- B The inferior turbinate
- C The part of the ethmoid with its middle and superior turbinates
- D The perpendicular plate of the palatine bone
- E The medial pterygoid plate

254 **Parapharyngeal abscess:**
- A Usually occurs as a complication of tonsillitis
- B Trismus occurs because of involvement of the medial pterygoid muscle
- C The neck is usually tender below the angle of the mandible
- D The tonsil may be pushed medially
- E Immediate surgical drainage is required

255 **Foreign bodies in the external auditory canal:**
- A Are commonest in children
- B Live insects should be removed with forceps
- C A postaural incision may be required for removal in some cases
- D Forceps should be used to remove round and smooth objects
- E Vegetable foreign bodies should be removed by syringing

256 **The orbit:**
- A The optic canal perforates the greater wing of the sphenoid
- B The maxilla forms part of its lateral wall
- C The anterior ethmoidal foramen is at the junction of the orbital plate of the maxilla and the orbital plate of the ethmoid
- D Division of superior cervical sympathetic nerve fibres results in ptosis
- E The superior orbital fissure leads into the pterygopalatine fossa

94 Answers

251 A T There are appreciable numbers of lymphocytes in thoracic duct lymph.
  B T
  C F Lymph contains clotting factors and will clot on standing *in vitro*.
  D F This is the fate of non-water-soluble fats.
  E T Because of the presence of chylomicrons – very large lipoprotein complexes – which enter the circulation via the lymphatic ducts.

252 A T A perforation of the tympanic membrane is the sole abnormality.
  B F No stapes superstructure is present, merely a mobile footplate.
  C T The stapedial footplate is fixed.
  D F This would be a 'type 3'.
  E T A lever mechanism is re-established between the tympanic membrane and the oval window, while the normal lateral dimensions of the tympanum are maintained.

253 A T The bony lateral nasal wall is made up of the nasal surface of the
  B T maxilla antero-inferiorly and the perpendicular plate of the palatine
  C T bone posteriorly. The inferior turbinate overlies these bones
  D T inferiorly. Most of the superior part is formed by part of the ethmoid
  E F bone with its middle and superior turbinates.

254 A T But may also complicate infection of a lower wisdom tooth.
  B T The medial pterygoid muscle contributes to the lateral wall of the parapharyngeal space.
  C T
  D T But not always, and it may appear normal.
  E F Intravenous antibiotics should be administered for the first 24–48 h following the onset of symptoms. Unless the response is dramatic, drainage should be carried out.

255 A T They are not uncommon in subnormal adults.
  B F They should be killed with surgical spirit and then removed.
  C T When there is a large and impacted object in the deep meatus.
  D F They may then slip deeper into the meatus during attempts at removal.
  E F They may be hygroscopic and swell if moistened.

256 A F It is situated within the lesser wing of the sphenoid.
  B F The lateral wall is formed by the zygoma and the greater wing of the sphenoid.
  C F It is situated between the orbital plate of the ethmoid and the orbital plate of the frontal bone.
  D T Due to paralysis of levator palpebrae superioris.
  E F The inferior orbital fissure does this. The superior orbital fissure leads into the middle cranial fossa.

257 **Metastatic carcinoma of the nose and sinuses:**
  A   Is rare when compared with primary tumours in this region
  B   The most common metastasis occurring in the maxilla is from a primary in the bronchus
  C   A frequent first symptom is epistaxis
  D   Metastases from renal cell carcinoma may be worth treating aggressively
  E   The overall survival is very poor

258 **Thyrotoxicosis:**
  A   Is more common in females
  B   Patients express a preference for cold environments
  C   Causes atrial fibrillation
  D   Appetite is increased
  E   Weight increases

259 **Loudness recruitment:**
  A   Is measured by performing speech audiometry
  B   Occurs more frequently in disorders of the cochlea
  C   Is a useful investigation in a complete unilateral deafness
  D   May be investigated by measurement of the stapedius reflex level
  E   A loudness balance test exhibiting loudness reversal always indicates a neural lesion

260 **The digastric muscle:**
  A   The posterior belly is longer than the anterior belly
  B   The anterior belly is attached to the superior genial tubercle on the mandible
  C   The motor nerve supply of the anterior belly is from the pharyngeal plexus
  D   The posterior belly is supplied by the facial nerve
  E   Elevates the hyoid bone

261 **Nasal malignant melanoma:**
  A   Accounts for approximately 1% of all cases of malignant melanoma
  B   Commonly presents with epistaxis
  C   Frequently presents with nasal obstruction
  D   Always appears as a dark brown or black lesion
  E   Invariably produces bone erosion

262 **Drugs used in respiratory disease:**
  A   Sodium cromoglycate is a bronchodilator
  B   Salbutamol is a selective stimulant of $beta_2$-adrenoceptors
  C   Codeine is used as an expectorant
  D   Candidiasis can occur following oral administration of inhaled steroids
  E   Terbutaline is a non-selective beta-stimulant

257   A   T
      B   F   The commonest is from renal cell carcinoma, followed by breast and lung.
      C   T   Nasal obstruction and deformity also occur.
      D   T   Resection of a solitary metastasis may occasionally be curative.
      E   T

258   A   T   About 8 times more common.
      B   T   As opposed to patients with hypothyroidism who express a preference for warmth.
      C   T   A frequent cause behind ischaemic heart disease and myocardial infarction.
      D   T
      E   F   Despite the increased appetite, weight usually decreases.

259   A   F   It is usually measured by performing alternative binaural loudness balances (Fowler's test).
      B   T   Thus helping to locate the site of the lesion.
      C   F   There must be at least some hearing present in both ears.
      D   T   It can also be assessed by measuring the loudness discomfort level and by Békésy and evoked response audiometry.
      E   T   A neural lesion – as opposed to a sensory lesion – causes a much severer impairment of speech discrimination for any level of pure tone threshold loss.

260   A   T
      B   F   It is attached at the digastric fossa on the base of the mandible.
      C   F   It is supplied by the mylohyoid branch of the inferior alveolar nerve, itself a branch of the mandibular nerve.
      D   T   Branches are given to the posterior belly of digastric and to stylohyoid before the nerve enters the parotid gland.
      E   T   It also depresses the mandible.

261   A   T
      B   T
      C   T   Nasal obstruction and epistaxis are the commonest features.
      D   F   Some are amelanotic and not pigmented.
      E   F   This is uncommon. Wide surgical excision is the treatment of choice giving a 5-year survival rate of 30%.

262   A   F   Sodium cromoglycate stabilizes sensitized mast cells and inhibits the release of bronchoconstrictor agents.
      B   T   Causing relaxation of bronchial smooth muscle and stabilization of mast cells.
      C   F   Codeine is used as a cough suppressant.
      D   T   But not as frequently as following systemic administration.
      E   F   Terbutaline is a selective $beta_2$-stimulant and acts in a similar fashion to salbutamol.

263 **Wegener's granulomatosis:**
A   Has only three basic nasal types
B   Does not cause nasal pain
C   Does not cause arthralgia
D   Is classically diagnosed by nasal biopsy
E   Is treated by cyclophosphamide and steroids

264 **Postcricoid carcinoma:**
A   Is usually visible on indirect laryngoscopy
B   Associated signs may be visible on indirect laryngoscopy
C   Laryngeal crepitus may be lost
D   Barium swallow is not a useful investigation
E   In the presence of homolateral involved mobile lymph glands, surgery is the treatment of choice

265 **Tympanosclerosis:**
A   Can affect the tympanic membrane as a direct consequence of grommet insertion
B   Tympanic membrane mobility may be impaired
C   Only affects the tympanic membrane
D   Plaques are vascularized
E   Of the tympanic membrane occurs in its middle fibrous layer

266 **The scalp:**
A   Has an abundance of sebaceous glands
B   Its blood vessels lie in the subaponeurotic layer
C   Has the richest cutaneous blood supply in the body
D   Venous drainage is not entirely to the superficial veins
E   Its periosteal layer is a continuous sheet over the skull

267 **Perennial non-allergic rhinitis:**
A   Presentation becomes more frequent with increasing age
B   Is associated with an increased sensitivity to histamine and metacholine nasal challenge
C   May be divided into two specific syndromes on the basis of nasal secretion eosinophil counts
D   Is not associated with nasal polyposis
E   Response is poor or absent to topical nasal steroids

263 A F To make the diagnosis there must be lung and/or renal involvement. There are, however, two distinct patterns of nasal involvement – one where nasal features predominate and the other occurring as part of a systemic disturbance.
     B F Pain is associated with nasal crusting and destruction.
     C F The 'systemic' disease causes anaemia, weakness, pallor, night sweats and migratory arthralgia.
     D T
     E T This is the treatment of choice but azathioprine and metronidazole may also be used.

264 A F It is most unusual to visualize the tumour if it is restricted to the postcricoid area.
     B T Pooling of saliva in the pyriform fossa and reduced or absent homolateral vocal cord mobility should arouse one's suspicions of this lesion.
     C T This is frequently the case.
     D F The lower limit of the neoplasm would be visualized and this may be the only means of assessing it. This helps to determine the most appropriate method of pharyngeal repair, if surgical intervention is to be considered.
     E T Radiotherapy will only cure 5% of such patients.

265 A T Although not the sole cause, tympanosclerosis is frequently seen over the site of a previous grommet insertion.
     B T Movement is invariably reduced and not uncommonly absent.
     C F It may also affect any one of several sites within the middle ear.
     D F They are avascular.
     E T When the tympanum is affected, the tympanosclerotic plaques are located between the mucosa and periosteum.

266 A T Hence the frequent abundance of sebaceous cysts in this area.
     B F They are deep to the skin in the subcutaneous connective tissue layer.
     C T
     D T There are numerous emissary veins piercing the skull.
     E F The periosteum adheres to the suture lines of the skull. Thus collections of blood or pus beneath this layer outline the affected bone.

267 A T Although allergic rhinitis is more common in childhood and most patients with allergic perennial rhinitis have an allergic history as a child. Perennial non-allergic rhinitis tends to present in adulthood.
     B T The nose is hyper-reactive in perennial non-allergic rhinitis.
     C T An eosinophilic group (one third) and a non-eosinophilic group (two thirds).
     D F 30% of patients in the eosinophilic group have nasal polyposis. The occurrence of polypi in other varieties of chronic rhinitis is merely coincidental.
     E F Those in the eosinophilic group show an excellent response. About 40% of patients in the non-eosinophilic group also respond favourably and the remainder obtain good control with ipratropium bromide.

268 **Features of acute uncomplicated bacterial tonsillitis include:**
A A positive Paul–Bunnell test
B Dysphagia
C Abdominal pain
D Displacement of one tonsil towards the midline
E Otalgia

269 **Postoperative facial paralysis:**
A The ear should be explored immediately if the paralysis is immediate and complete
B Occurs more commonly when using the electric drill than with a hammer and gouge
C If nerve trauma is suspected, a 48 h delay in re-exploration is of little significance
D May occur following a stapedectomy
E A delayed partial paralysis should usually be re-explored

270 **Normal bacterial flora include:**
A Streptococci in the nasal cavity
B Streptococci in the mouth
C Yeasts in the stomach
D Spirochaetes in the mouth
E Staphylococci on the skin

271 **The mandibular division of the trigeminal nerve:**
A Is separated from tensor palati by the otic ganglion
B Gives off two branches from a short trunk and then divides into an anterior group and a posterior group of branches
C The branches of the anterior group are all motor except one sensory branch – the lingual nerve
D The branches of the posterior group are all sensory except one motor branch – the nerve to masseter
E Usually two deep temporal branches enter the temporalis muscle anteriorly

272 **Nasal septoplasty:**
A A full transfixion incision may lead to tip collapse
B Separation of the upper lateral cartilages from the nasal septum does not tend to lead to a supratip depression
C A submucosal resection of the nasal septum (SMR) is not included as a part of the operation
D Differs from a Killian SMR in that there is preservation, rather than excision, of nasal septal cartilage
E Has a greater risk of cartilage necrosis than does an SMR

268 A F This would indicate the presence of glandular fever.
     B T This is often severe.
     C T Mesenteric adenitis is not uncommon in children.
     D F This would indicate the presence of a peritonsillar abscess or, less commonly, a parapharyngeal abscess.
     E T Presumably referred via the glossopharyngeal nerve.

269 A F At least 4 h should elapse to enable the effect of any local anaesthesia used for periaural infiltration to wear off, as long as the surgeon is not aware of any iatrogenic damage.
     B F The hammer and gouge are more likely to displace bony fragments towards the nerve.
     C F Early surgery offers the best results.
     D T Especially during a 'drill out' procedure for otosclerosis.
     E F Packing should be loosened and antibiotics prescribed but re-exploration is seldom required.

270 A F But staphylococci are considered as normal flora, affecting 30% of the population.
     B T
     C F The stomach is normally sterile.
     D T Other normal flora in the mouth include staphylococci, yeasts, anaerobic and enteric bacteria, and Actinomyces and Haemophilus species.
     E T

271 A T Just below the foramen ovale.
     B T These two branches are the nervus spinosus to the dura and the nerve to the medial pterygoid.
     C F The sole sensory nerve of the anterior group is the buccal nerve.
     D F The sole motor nerve of the posterior group is the mylohyoid branch of the inferior alveolar nerve.
     E T Hence the muscle can be mobilized posteriorly and used to obliterate the middle ear and mastoid.

272 A T Scarring may cause tip collapse and a hemitransfixion incision is usually recommended.
     B F Supratip depression tends to occur in the long-term unless the upper lateral cartilages are approximated to the nasal septum with absorbable sutures. Unless a septoplasty is performed through an external incision, such a repair is not possible.
     C F All septoplasties invariably involve some resection of bone and cartilage.
     D T An SMR attempts to remove the deformity whereas a septoplasty attempts to correct it.
     E F Cartilage necrosis is not usually a problem in septoplasty, as long as blood is not allowed to accumulate. A perforation in one flap avoids this complication. Most surgeons find that elevating the flaps allows such perforations to occur with ease!

273 **Anomalies of the thyroglossal tract:**
 A A lingual thyroid may represent the only thyroid tissue present
 B A thyroglossal cyst occurs more commonly above the hyoid
 C When occurring in the subhyoid position, a thyroglossal cyst is always situated in the midline
 D A thyroglossal cyst should invariably be excised
 E A thyroglossal fistula is never congenital

274 **Audiometric tests:**
 A Abnormal adaptation demonstrated by a tone decay test implies a neural lesion
 B Tone decay occurs in normal hearing ears
 C In Békésy audiometry the patient traces out his or her own threshold
 D The acoustic (stapedius) reflex is useful in the investigation of a facial palsy
 E Impedance tests may aid in the diagnosis of a glomus tumour

275 **Contents of the infratemporal fossa include:**
 A The maxillary nerve
 B The mandibular nerve
 C The facial nerve
 D The lateral pterygoid muscle
 E The medial pterygoid muscle

276 **Rhinosporidiosis:**
 A Is caused by *Rhinosporidium seeberi*
 B The organism can readily be cultured on Sabouraud's medium
 C Infection is caused by inhaling infected dust
 D The nasal disease develops into a painless polypoidal lesion filling the nose
 E Effective treatment is by complete surgical excision

277 **Metronidazole:**
 A Is active against *Staphylococcus aureus*
 B Is effective against Bacteroides species
 C Is used to treat chronic sinusitis
 D Alcohol is contraindicated during therapy
 E Causes hyperkalaemia when taken in large doses

278 **Complications following head and neck surgery:**
 A The intracranial pressure rises three-fold following ligation of one internal jugular vein
 B A chylous fistula occurs more commonly following left-sided neck surgery
 C A seroma occurs more frequently within the first 24 h after surgery
 D The presence of diabetes mellitus may prevent adequate wound healing
 E Deep vein thrombosis occurs in approximately 5% of cases operated on for malignancy

273 A T It usually forms a rounded swelling at the foramen caecum.
     B F It occurs most commonly beneath the hyoid, followed by the region of the thyroid cartilage.
     C T Such cysts are always in the midline. However, cysts occurring in the region of the thyroid cartilage are not uncommonly off-centre.
     D T Infection is usually inevitable because the cyst contains lymphatic tissue which communicates with the lymph nodes of the neck.
     E T It follows infection or inadequate removal of a thyroglosssal cyst.

274 A T This is the usual implication but abnormal adaptation may still occur in the presence of a cochlear lesion.
     B T But it should be less than 15 dB.
     C T Performed to both a continuous and a pulsed stimulus.
     D T If the nerve to the stapedius is not functioning the muscle will not reflexly contract.
     E T The compliance needle will oscillate at maximum sensitivity in time with the pulse. The oscillations are damped when the ipsilateral carotid is compressed.

275 A F The infratemporal fossa is situated beneath the skull-base, between
     B T the lateral wall of the pharynx and the ascending ramus of the
     C F mandible. It contains, in addition, the maxillary artery and the
     D T pterygoid venous plexus.
     E T

276 A T
     B F Sabouraud's medium is for fungi. *Rhinosporidium seeberi* has not been grown on any culture medium.
     C F Infection occurs following immersion in contaminated water.
     D T Having initially commenced as a flat and sessile lesion.
     E T There is no effective medical treatment.

277 A F
     B T It is also effective against Fusiform bacteria, Clostridia, anaerobic cocci and some protozoa.
     C T Anaerobic organisms are frequently implicated in the aetiology of chronic sinusitis.
     D T There exists the possibility of a disulfiram-like reaction, i.e. the inhibition of alcohol dehydrogenase.
     E F

278 A T The increase becomes five-fold when both are simultaneously ligated.
     B T The thoracic duct is on the left side.
     C F Seromas are more likely to occur in the first 48 h following the removal of the drains.
     D T Good preoperative control is required. Other factors delaying wound healing include poor nutritional status, anaemia, uraemia, hypothyroidism, neoplasia, previous radiotherapy and infection.
     E F Its occurrence is extremely unusual following major head and neck surgery and its incidence is less than 1%.

279 **Physiology of hearing:**
A   Only 'piston-like' movement of the stapes occurs in the oval window
B   The mallear arm of the ossicular chain lever system is longer than the incudal arm by a ratio of 1.3:1
C   The ratio of the areas of the tympanic membrane and the oval window is 14:1
D   A travelling sound wave along the basilar membrane is solely longitudinal
E   All auditory nerve fibres fire at least to some degree when stimulated by sound of any intensity

280 **The floor of the mouth:**
A   Consists mainly of mylohyoid
B   The submandibular duct opens into the mouth opposite the second lower premolar
C   The lingual nerve enters the mouth by passing below the inferior border of the superior constrictor
D   The glossopharyngeal nerve is motor to the intrinsic lingual muscles
E   The sublingual gland drains all of its secretions into the sublingual papilla

281 **The nasal trigeminal afferents play a role in:**
A   The afferent pathway of sneezing
B   The control of respiration
C   Nasal sensation of airflow
D   Nasal pain
E   Reflexes involving nasal resistance to airflow

282 **Nasopharyngeal angiofibroma:**
A   May arise from the posterior nasal cavity
B   May reach the anterior nares
C   Biopsy should be obtained prior to undertaking any treatment
D   Tends to appear as a round and lobulated firm red swelling
E   Forms 0.5% of all head and neck neoplasms

283 **Auricular haematoma:**
A   Occurs more commonly in the elderly
B   The single most important principle of management is drainage of the haematoma
C   A 'cauliflower ear' may follow delayed treatment
D   Most occur posteriorly on the pinna
E   The haematoma is within cartilage

279 A F Rocking movements also occur about longitudinal and transverse axes at different sound intensities.
     B T
     C T Thus the overall ratio of the middle ear transformer mechanism is 14 × 1.3 = 18.3.
     D F A transverse deformation of the basilar membrane also occurs.
     E F Each auditory nerve fibre has an optimum stimulus frequency and beyond certain frequency ranges the nerve fibre will not fire at any intensity.

280 A T Above this muscle is the mouth and below it is the neck.
     B F It opens immediately lateral to the frenulum linguae as a small elevation – the sublingual papilla.
     C T At its attachment to the mandible.
     D F The intrinsic lingual muscles are supplied by the hypoglossal nerve.
     E F Half of the sublingual ducts open directly into the submandibular duct.

281 A F The pathway for sneezing runs in the Vidian nerve. If it is cut, stimulation of the nasal mucosa does not produce sneezing.
     B T It is thought that the nasal trigeminal afferents help in the fine control of respiration.
     C T
     D T
     E T

282 A T It may arise from the region of the sphenopalatine foramen.
     B T It is frequently very large.
     C F Biopsy should not be obtained because of the risk of excessive bleeding. Once the tumour is suspected clinically, further confirmation is obtained by simple radiography, CT scanning and angiography.
     D T
     E T

283 A F It is most prevalent in young and active individuals.
     B F Of equal importance is obliteration of the subperichondrial space, either by pressure or by suction drainage.
     C T Fibrosis and scarring occur and the cartilage becomes thickened and irregular.
     D F Most occur anteriorly because, on this aspect of the pinna, the skin does not have the ability to slide and so the shearing produced between skin and cartilage leads to haemorrhage.
     E F It is in the subperichondrial space.

284 **The fascia of the neck:**
- A The deep cervical fascia lies deep to platysma
- B The deep cervical fascia splits to invest trapezius
- C The anterior layer of the pretracheal fascia splits to enclose the thyroid gland
- D The pretracheal fascia splits around the infrahyoid strap muscles
- E The constituents of the ansa cervicalis are embedded in the carotid sheath

285 **Polyarteritis nodosa:**
- A Is a necrotizing vasculitis of small and medium-sized arteries
- B May present in the nose with epistaxis
- C Tends to progress to arthritis, myopathy and renal failure
- D Causes sudden deafness
- E Causes non-specific nasal lesions

286 **Thyroiditis:**
- A de Quervain's thyroiditis has a viral aetiology
- B In Riedel's thyroiditis there is no goitre
- C Hashimoto's disease is associated with hyperthyroidism
- D Hashimoto's thyroiditis is an autoimmune disorder
- E A subtotal thyroidectomy is the usual treatment for Hashimoto's thyroiditis

287 **Intranasal antrostomy:**
- A The antrostomy should be extended as far forwards as possible
- B The antrostomy should be extended as high as possible
- C The antrostomy should be extended as low as possible
- D The antrostomy should be extended as far posteriorly as possible
- E Haemorrhage from the sphenopalatine artery is not an uncommon problem during this operation

288 **The utricle and saccule:**
- A The saccule is the smaller of the two
- B The saccule joins the duct of the cochlea by the saccular duct
- C The utricular duct connects the utricle to the endolymphatic duct
- D The membranous semicircular ducts open into the utricle by six separate openings
- E The saccule may be no more than 0.4 mm from the stapes footplate

289 **Steroids, when used to control the inflammation of allergy:**
- A Reduce prostaglandin synthesis by blocking cyclo-oxygenase
- B Reduce prostaglandin synthesis by blocking phospholipase
- C Reduce the release and synthesis of inflammatory mediators by reducing the influx of calcium ions into the mast cell
- D Reduce the recruitment of eosinophils
- E Are particularly effective at reducing the late phase of the allergic response

284   A T
     B T It also splits to invest sternomastoid.
     C T
     D F It lies deep to them.
     E T Along with the common and internal carotid arteries, the internal jugular vein and the vagus nerve.

285   A T It is a systemic vasculitis.
     B F It tends to present insidiously with minor complaints, before progressing to become systemic.
     C T
     D T
     E T Although the nose is frequently involved in the vasculitis.

286   A T Possibly a mumps virus.
     B F The goitre is unilateral or bilateral and is usually woody-hard and fixed.
     C T Initially only, but hypothyroidism is inevitable.
     D T Histological examination shows the presence of many lymphocytes.
     E F Treatment is with thyroxine. Thyroidectomy is required only rarely for cosmesis.

287   A T Care should be taken not to extend to the anterior surface of the maxilla.
     B F If the antrostomy is too high the nasolacrimal duct may be damaged.
     C T The antrostomy should be level with the nasal floor.
     D F
     E T The antrostomy should not go too far posteriorly, otherwise damage to the sphenopalatine artery and severe epistaxis are likely.

288   A T It lies in a depression below and in front of the utricle.
     B F The ductus reuniens joins the two.
     C T
     D F There are five separate openings as one limb of the posterior and one limb of the superior semicircular canals join to form the crus commune.
     E T And the surface of the utricle as near as 0.65 mm.

289   A F Steroids interfere with the enzyme phospholipase A_2 which liberates
     B T arachidonic acid from cell membrane phospholipid.
     C T They do this by causing the synthesis of a protein, lipocortin, which inhibits the enzyme. Calcium ions are essential for the operation of phospholipase A_2.
     D T By inhibiting mast cell degranulation and liberation of ECF-A (Eosinophilic chemotactic factor of anaphylaxis).
     E T

290 **Nasopharyngeal carcinoma:**
   A Accounts for 98% of malignant lesions of the nasopharynx
   B Anaplastic carcinoma is the most common histological grading
   C Is more commonly non-keratinizing
   D The axilla and mediastinum should be included in radiotherapy fields as a matter of course
   E Anaplastic carcinoma frequently presents as a large exophytic lesion

291 **The cerebral hemispheres:**
   A The basal ganglia are masses of white matter
   B The precentral area of the frontal lobe is concerned with motor function
   C The auditory centre receives its blood supply from the middle cerebral artery
   D Parkinsonism would result following disease of the globus pallidus
   E The thalamus forms the lateral wall of the third ventricle

292 **Vestibular function:**
   A The vestibular sensory epithelium and the muscle, joint and skin sense receptors are the principal sensory sources for balance
   B The cupulae of the semicircular canals respond to angular acceleration
   C The maculae of the utricle and saccule respond to angular acceleration
   D The slow component of nystagmus is of vestibular origin
   E Loss of one labyrinth results in spontaneous nystagmus towards the affected ear

293 **Leukaemia:**
   A Epistaxis occurs in the more chronic forms
   B Acute myeloid leukaemia is the most common acute leukaemia in adults
   C Acute lymphoblastic leukaemia is the most common acute leukaemia in children
   D Epistaxis is not an uncommon presenting feature of acute leukaemia
   E Lesions affecting the throat are uncommon manifestations of acute leukaemia

294 **Congenital disorders of the larynx:**
   A A bifid epiglottis is invariably asymptomatic
   B Haemangiomas of the larynx are associated with haemangiomas of the skin of the head and neck region
   C Chondromas have a predilection for the supraglottis
   D Bilateral vocal cord paralysis is associated with hydrocephalus
   E Congenital laryngeal clefts are situated posteriorly

290   A   T
       B   T
       C   T Most squamous carcinomas are non-keratinizing.
       D   T These lymph node groups are not infrequently involved in the disease.
       E   T

291   A   F They are grey matter and comprise the corpus striatum, the claustrum and the amygdala.
       B   T The postcentral area of the parietal lobe is concerned with sensory function.
       C   T This is the largest branch of the internal carotid artery.
       D   T Affecting the extrapyramidal pathways and resulting in disturbance of voluntary movement and muscle tone.
       E   T The thalamus contains nuclei of the sensory tracts.

292   A   F Visual stimuli are of equal importance.
       B   T
       C   F They respond to linear acceleration of the head.
       D   T The rapid component depends upon cerebral cortical adjustment.
       E   F The fast component of the nystagmus would be towards the opposite side but, after several weeks, compensation does occur.

293   A   F Epistaxes occur much more frequently in the acute leukaemias.
       B   T
       C   T
       D   T
       E   F They are relatively common.

294   A   F In this rare condition, half of the epiglottis is frequently sucked into the glottis and obstructs the airway.
       B   T One should always be alert to this possible association.
       C   F They invariably present in the subglottis.
       D   T And the prognosis is poor. Unilateral vocal cord paralysis occurs more commonly and is usually the result of birth trauma.
       E   T The cleft passes through the posterior plate of the cricoid and some way down the trachea. They are notoriously difficult to diagnose.

295 **The nerve supply to:**
A   The maxillary antrum is derived solely from the maxillary nerve and its branches
B   The ethmoidal sinuses are derived solely from the ethmoidal nerves
C   The frontal sinus is derived solely from the ophthalmic nerves
D   The sphenoid sinus is derived solely from the ophthalmic nerve and its branches
E   The sphenoid sinus is derived from the maxillary nerve and its branches

296 **Laboratory temporal bone dissection:**
A   Is not an essential practice
B   The temporal bone should be secured with plaster of Paris
C   A general rule of dissection is to use the largest possible burr for a given area
D   Temporal bones need not include the petrous tip
E   Ideally, the microscope should closely resemble the unit used in the operating theatre

297 **In perennial rhinitis without chest symptoms:**
A   The nose is hypersensitive to metacholine challenge
B   The nose is hypersensitive to histamine challenge
C   The bronchi are not hyper-reactive to histamine challenge
D   Nasal resistance values are, on average, higher than in the general population
E   Rhinomanometry is a useful diagnostic test

298 **Adenoid cystic carcinoma:**
A   Arises from minor salivary glands
B   Grows along perineural sheaths
C   Has a preference for the ethmoidal sinuses
D   Is very slow-growing
E   Has a high 5-year survival rate

299 **The tongue:**
A   Styloglossus draws the tongue forwards
B   The lingual nerve is motor to most of the lingual musculature
C   Contains some unstriated muscle
D   Is partly situated in the hypopharynx
E   The deep lingual vein can be visualized in the mouth

110   *Answers*

295   A T
      B F Branches of the maxillary nerve also supply the ethmoidal sinuses.
      C T
      D F
      E F The sphenoid sinus is supplied by branches of both the maxillary and
            ophthalmic nerves.

296   A F It is widely accepted that temporal bone dissection on a regular basis
            is a fundamental learning experience to the otologist.
      B F Although securing with plaster of Paris appears physiological, more
            knowledge is obtained if it is secured in a stainless steel bone holder
            with three-point fixation in order to allow for further inspection and
            repositioning during the course of the dissection.
      C T This is especially true when approaching areas where a burr could
            plunge through the dural plate or into a cavity.
      D F Each bone should include all the mastoid air cells, some of the
            squamous bone, the tympanic ring and the petrous tip, although
            dissection of the petrous apex is not relevant to most otologists.
      E T As should the instruments, in order to familiarize the surgeon with
            the instruments to be used during surgery.

297   A T
      B T In perennial rhinitis the nose is generally hyper-reactive.
      C F The nose is only one part of the respiratory tract and in perennial
            rhinitis, even in the absence of chest symptoms, the bronchi can be
            shown to be hyper-reactive.
      D T
      E F Although the mean nasal resistance values for individuals are higher
            in perennial rhinitis than normals, the degree of scatter of results is such
            that rhinomanometry cannot be used as a diagnostic test of perennial
            rhinitis.

298   A T
      B T
      C F Of the sinuses, the maxillary antrum is the commoner site.
      D T
      E F The tumour, although very slow-growing, tends to cause pulmonary
            metastases and the 5-year survival is only in the region of 10%.

299   A F It draws the tongue upwards and backwards.
      B F The lingual nerve carries sensory and secretomotor nerve fibres only.
      C F All of its muscle is striated.
      D F It is situated in the oropharynx and oral cavity.
      E T It can be seen through the mucous membrane lateral to the
            frenulum linguae.

300 **The middle ear:**
- A Communicates with the mastoid antrum through the aditus posteriorly
- B Communicates with the nasopharynx through the eustachian tube superiorly
- C The distance between the tympanic membrane and the promontory is 8 mm
- D The main body of the ossicles is situated in the epitympanic recess
- E The sinus tympani is that space immediately lateral to the descending portion of the facial nerve

301 **Sjögren's syndrome:**
- A Is diagnosed when the patient has two of the following: xerostomia, xerophthalmia and a connective tissue disease
- B Often produces salivary gland enlargement
- C Is commoner in men
- D Tends not to cause epistaxes
- E Tends not to cause nasal septal perforations

302 **Carcinoma of the pyriform fossa:**
- A Is usually visible on indirect laryngoscopy
- B Adenocarcinoma is the commonest histological type
- C Is associated with sideropenic dysphagia
- D Surgical excision would invariably also include a laryngectomy
- E Is the commonest site of the occurrence of a hypopharyngeal neoplasm

303 **The hyoid bone:**
- A The digastric muscle has an attachment
- B Ossification commences in the lesser cornua around birth
- C The lesser cornua are attached by their bases at the angle of the junction of the body and greater cornua
- D The middle constrictor arises from the greater cornu
- E Gives attachment to the investing layer of deep fascia

304 **Recurrent acute otitis media:**
- A Affects 10% of children in the first decade
- B May be hereditary
- C Allergy is the principal cause
- D Is associated with nasal polypi
- E Is associated with teething

305 **Nasal decongestants include:**
- A Pilocarpine
- B Prostaglandin E_2
- C Prostaglandin I_2 (prostacyclin)
- D Aspirin
- E Phenylpropanolamine

300   A   T
      B   F   This communication is anterior.
      C   F   It is nearer to 2 mm.
      D   T   This is the upward extension behind the roof of the external auditory meatus, also known as the attic.
      E   F   This is the facial recess. The sinus tympani lies medial to the facial nerve.

301   A   T
      B   T   Which may be bilateral and symmetrical.
      C   F   It is nine times commoner in women.
      D   F   Epistaxes occur in approximately 50%.
      E   F   Nasal crusting and drying precede nasal septal perforation.

302   A   T   Invariably.
      B   F   Most are squamous cell carcinomas.
      C   F   Sideropenic dysphagia (Paterson–Brown–Kelly syndrome) is associated with postcricoid carcinoma.
      D   T   Most agree that the operation of choice is a total laryngectomy and a partial or total pharyngectomy, plus a radical neck dissection if the regional lymph nodes are involved.
      E   T   Followed by postcricoid and the posterior hypopharyngeal wall.

303   A   F   Not directly, but its intermediate tendon is held beneath a fibrous ring attached near the lesser cornu.
      B   F   This occurs around puberty.
      C   T   They may occasionally be connected to the body of the hyoid by fibrous tissue.
      D   T   And also from the stylohyoid ligament.
      E   T   Hence there is no 'dewlap' as in cattle.

304   A   F   It affects only 1%.
      B   T   Some children certainly have an inherited susceptibility to such attacks.
      C   F   The chief cause is persistent infection within the upper respiratory tract.
      D   F   No such association is known.
      E   T   In some obscure way such an association exists.

305   A   F   Pilocarpine is a cholinomimetic agent and will congest the nose.
      B   T   Prostaglandin E_2 is a potent vasoconstrictor and will decongest the nose.
      C   F   Prostaglandin I_2 causes vasodilatation throughout the body, including the nose, and will cause nasal obstruction.
      D   F   Aspirin inhibits prostaglandin synthesis and causes nasal obstruction.
      E   T   Phenylpropanolamine is an α-receptor agonist causing nasal decongestion.

306 **Carcinoma of the nose and sinuses is associated with:**
A   Nickel refiners
B   Woodworkers
C   Cobblers
D   Snuff takers
E   Asbestos workers

307 **Nasal embryology:**
A   The medial components of the frontonasal process become the nasal septum
B   The developing nasal cavities are separated from the oral cavity by the bucconasal membrane
C   The nasal capsule becomes divided into upper and lower lateral and septal cartilages
D   The vomer ossifies from cartilage
E   The part of the ethmoid forming the cribriform plate has ossified by birth

308 **Auricular perichondritis:**
A   The ear is tender but not red
B   May follow an auricular haematoma
C   Perichondrium is especially susceptible to infection caused by *Pseudomonas aeruginosa*
D   Can occur following middle ear surgery
E   May follow otitis externa

309 **The following commonly cause acute bacterial sinusitis:**
A   *Streptococcus pneumoniae*
B   *Haemophilus influenzae*
C   *Branhamella catarrhalis*
D   *Staphylococcus aureus*
E   In at least 30% of cases anaerobic bacteria may be cultured

310 **Fistulae following head and neck surgery:**
A   Occur more commonly in the irradiated patient
B   A type 2 fistula is one in which there is no local healthy tissue and for repair both surfaces must be provided from a distance
C   A type 1 fistula requires for repair an outer covering from a distance
D   Disruption of the suture line is the commoner cause in the non-irradiated patient
E   Pharyngocutaneous fistulae occur after resection of buccal tumours

306 A T It appears that nickel refiners, rather than those working with nickel itself, are at risk.
     B T It is commoner in those exposed to fine particles of hardwood dust which have been heated by the use of high-speed woodworking machines (such as teak).
     C T The exact cause is not known.
     D F Those who chew tobacco are at risk from oral cancer.
     E F

307 A T Embryonic development of the nose starts in the third fetal week.
     B T
     C T By an ingrowth of connective tissue in the sixth fetal month.
     D F The vomer is formed from ossification in connective tissue existing on either side of the septal cartilage.
     E F That part of the ethmoid forming the cribriform plate remains fibrous until the third year. When it ossifies, it stabilizes the entire ethmoid complex.

308 A F The pinna is red and tender in the early stages.
     B T A good culture medium would then be present and further infection may be introduced during aspiration or incision.
     C T The appropriate antibiotic would then need to be instituted, preferably administered by the parenteral route.
     D T Following the injudicial placement of the incision or as a result of a meatoplasty.
     E T Especially furunculosis.

309 A T
     B T
     C T
     D T
     E F Anaerobic organisms can be cultured in only 10% of cases.

310 A T There is a greater likelihood of tissue necrosis.
     B F This would be a type 3 fistula.
     C F This describes a type 2 fistula. In a type 1 fistula both epithelial surfaces can be provided locally.
     D T Tissue necrosis is the principal cause in the irradiated patient.
     E F Orocutaneous fistulae are more likely to occur.

311 **The cutaneous nerve supply of the face, scalp and neck:**
- A The external nasal nerve, a branch of the nasociliary division of the ophthalmic nerve, supplies the tip of the nose
- B The upper lip is supplied by the buccal branch of the mandibular nerve
- C The supra-orbital branch of the maxillary nerve supplies the occiput
- D The lacrimal branch of the ophthalmic nerve supplies the lateral part of the upper eyelid
- E The mental branch of the inferior alveolar division of the mandibular nerve is sensory to the area over the thyroid cartilage

312 **Herpes zoster oticus:**
- A Implies previous exposure to the chickenpox virus
- B Pain is a common feature
- C A maculopapular rash occurs frequently
- D Vesicles occur in the distribution of other cranial nerves beside the facial nerve
- E The prognosis for full recovery of facial nerve function is poor compared to that of Bell's palsy

313 **Topical nasal decongestants:**
- A Are alpha-adrenoceptor agonists
- B May be safely used for periods of several months
- C Effectively reduce nasal resistance to airflow in normal subjects
- D May be used to help differentiate between mucosal swelling and skeletal stenosis
- E Tend to increase nasal hyper-reactivity

314 **Nasopharyngeal carcinoma:**
- A In a lympho-epithelioma both the lymphocytes and the epithelial components are malignant
- B A substantial number arise from the fossa of Rosenmüller
- C The middle cranial fossa is invaded mostly via the jugular foramen
- D An *en bloc* radical neck dissection will remove all involved lymph nodes
- E If cranial nerve palsies are present on presentation, the prognosis is almost hopeless

315 **The nasopharynx:**
- A The eustachian tube opens into its lateral wall 2 cm behind the inferior turbinate
- B The floor of the fossa of Rosenmüller is closely related to the carotid canal
- C Is cuboidal in shape
- D Has both transverse and vertical diameters of 4 cm
- E The fossa of Rosenmüller may exceed 1 cm in depth

116   Answers

311 A T And also the skin of the alae and the nasal vestibule.
     B F It is supplied by the infra-orbital division of the maxillary nerve.
     C F This area is supplied by the greater occipital nerve (C2 and C3).
     D T But, when absent, its place is taken by the zygomaticotemporal branch of the maxillary nerve.
     E F This area is supplied by the cervical plexus.

312 A T As occurs with systemic herpes zoster infection (shingles).
     B T This usually precedes the appearance of the facial paralysis.
     C F A vesicular rash is invariably present over the tympanic membrane, in the external auditory meatus and on the pinna.
     D T They occur, not infrequently, over the palate.
     E T Severe otalgia at the outset is thought to herald a poor prognosis.

313 A T The two common topical nasal decongestants are xylometazoline and oxymetazoline, and both are alpha-sympathetic agonists. Isoprenaline is a beta-sympathetic receptor agonist.
     B F After approximately 2 weeks, rhinitis medicamentosa occurs. This condition is associated with a reduction in the number of x-receptors. x-Receptor agonists facilitate degranulation of mast cells.
     C T These agents reduce nasal resistance to airflow objectively.
     D T By rhinomanometry.
     E T

314 A F Lympho-epithelioma simply describes the histological picture of carcinoma containing a large number of normal lymphocytes.
     B T
     C F The middle cranial fossa is usually entered by the tumour extending along the carotid artery via the carotid canal.
     D F A radical neck dissection to include *en bloc* removal of metastases would have to include the nodes of Rouvière and the parapharyngeal lymphatics. Technically, this is not feasible.
     E T

315 A F This distance is 1 cm.
     B T The roof of the fossa of Rosenmüller is related to the foramen lacerum and its floor is directly related to the carotid canal.
     C T
     D T Its anteroposterior diameter is 2 cm.
     E T The fossa of Rosenmüller shows wide variation between individuals.

316 **The vestibular nerve:**
   A   The superior vestibular nerve supplies the posterior semicircular canal
   B   The inferior vestibular nerve supplies the macula of the utricle
   C   In the internal auditory meatus most of the vestibular nerve lies above the cochlear nerve
   D   The singular nerve supplies the posterior semicircular canal
   E   In the pons and medulla there are four vestibular nuclei on each side

317 **Syphilis:**
   A   Its primary lesion, the chancre, commonly involves the nose
   B   The secondary lesions of syphilis commonly affect the nose
   C   The typical nasal syphilitic lesion is extensive cartilaginous and bony destruction
   D   The number of new cases of syphilis in the USA is double the number of new cases of rubella in any given period of time
   E   Nasal syphilis is treated with high doses of systemic penicillin

318 **Tonsillectomy:**
   A   Bleeding is less troublesome when the operation is performed under local anaesthesia
   B   Draffin's bipods are the best apparatus for securing the position of the mouth gag
   C   Tonsil dissection commences at the upper pole
   D   Bleeding is less troublesome when the operation is performed using the Popper guillotine
   E   Dissection should take place within the substance of the tonsil

319 **The maxillary artery:**
   A   With the superficial temporal artery is a terminal division of the internal carotid artery
   B   Is more anteriorly situated than the maxillary nerve in the pterygopalatine fossa
   C   Usually has five branches
   D   The accessory meningeal branch enters the cranial cavity through the foramen spinosum
   E   The third part of the artery gives branches which accompany the branches of the pterygopalatine ganglion

320 **The tympanic membrane:**
   A   The incudostapedial joint may be visible through a normal tympanic membrane
   B   Is always normal in otitis externa
   C   Is likely to bulge in secretory otitis media
   D   Eustachian tube dysfunction results in its retraction
   E   Usually exhibits a reduction in mobility with ossicular discontinuity

316   A F This is supplied by the inferior vestibular nerve.
     B F This is supplied by the superior vestibular nerve.
     C T The cochlear nerve is situated medially and inferiorly within the internal auditory canal.
     D T Piercing the lamina cribrosa at the foramen singulare.
     E T Secondary central pathways pass from the vestibular nuclei to the vestibulospinal tract, from the medial longitudinal bundle to the extrinsic ocular muscles and to the cerebellum.

317   A F
     B F Primary and secondary syphilis are both rare in the nose.
     C T Typical nasal syphilis is tertiary and produces combined osseous and bony destruction.
     D T 27 000 new cases were reported in 1980.
     E T As is the treatment for the disease affecting any part of the body.

318   A T Although this is rarely practised in the UK.
     B F Not necessarily. There are many different techniques and each surgeon prefers his or her own.
     C T Which is then mobilized towards the lower pole.
     D T This has a crushing and cutting action in contrast to the Ballenger guillotine which only has a cutting action.
     E F It is carried out in the peritonsillar plane and the substance of the tonsil should not be entered.

319   A F They are the two terminal divisions of the external carotid artery.
     B T This becomes evident during a transantral Vidian nerve neurectomy.
     C F There are at least 15 branches, five from each of three parts, before, on and beyond the lateral pterygoid muscle.
     D F It passes through the foramen ovale.
     E T Mostly supplying the nasal cavity.

320   A T As may the stapedius muscle and the chorda tympani nerve.
     B F It is affected, not uncommonly, by the disease process causing the otitis externa.
     C F The tympanic membrane would, more commonly, be retracted.
     D T Because a potential vacuum develops in the middle ear.
     E F Its mobility is invariably increased.

321 **Non-allergic rhinitis may be caused or exacerbated by:**
   A   Beta-adrenoceptor antagonists
   B   Methyldopa
   C   Reserpine
   D   Barbiturates
   E   Chlorpromazine

322 **Fibrous dysplasia (ossifying fibroma):**
   A   May form part of Alport's syndrome
   B   Occurs in the first 20 years of life
   C   Typically produces painless facial swelling
   D   Radiology will usually differentiate it from osteogenic sarcoma
   E   Should be operated upon at an early stage in order to prevent the occurrence of malignant change

323 **The ethmoidal air cells:**
   A   The ethmoidal labyrinth often extends beyond the limits of the ethmoid bone
   B   The agger nasi cell occurs in 50% of individuals
   C   Anterior ethmoidal cells are defined as those that drain into the infundibulum of the middle meatus
   D   Middle ethmoidal cells are defined as those that drain into the region of the bulla ethmoidalis
   E   Posterior ethmoidal cells are defined as those that drain into the superior meatus

324 **Otic barotrauma:**
   A   Boyle's law states that the volume of a fixed mass of gas is directly proportional to its pressure
   B   Will occur during ascent in an aeroplane
   C   The eustachian tube opens passively to the passage of air from the middle ear
   D   The eustachian tube becomes 'locked' when the pressure differential on either side of the tympanic membrane exceeds 90 mmHg
   E   May be prevented by sucking sweets during aeroplane descent

325 **Submucosal resection of the nasal septum (SMR):**
   A   The incision is made parallel to and 1 cm posterior to the anterior edge of the nasal septum
   B   Dorsal and anterior cartilage struts should be left in place
   C   The maxillary crest should not be removed
   D   The maxillary crest may be in-fractured with little risk of it redeforming
   E   A torn mucoperichondrial flap on one side should be meticulously sutured

321 A T Beta-blocking drugs can cause severe rhinorrhoea.
  B T Methyldopa reduces sympathetic tone and thus increases nasal resistance to airflow.
  C T As for methyldopa.
  D F
  E F Neither barbiturates nor chlorpromazine have been implicated in vasomotor rhinitis.

322 A F Fibrous dysplasia ranges from a local monostotic lesion, usually of the maxilla, to diffuse polyostotic lesions associated with Albright's syndrome.
  B T
  C T
  D T
  E F The lesion is not malignant and major facial remodelling should be postponed until growth has ceased. Biopsy material should be obtained, however, in order to establish a diagnosis.

323 A T The ethmoidal air cells frequently extend into any of the bones adjacent to the ethmoid, such as the nasal bones, the sphenoid and the maxilla.
  B F The agger nasi cell occurs in 80% of the population.
  C T
  D T
  E T

324 A F They are inversely proportional.
  B F Problems occur during descent when the dilator muscles of the eustachian tube must work actively to enable air to enter the middle ear space.
  C T As would occur during ascent in an aircraft.
  D T The tympanic membrane would probably then perforate.
  E T Because the increased amount of swallowing will allow the eustachian tube to open more times than at rest.

325 A F The incision should be parallel to the caudal end of the septal cartilage and 5 mm posterior to it.
  B T In order to provide nasal support. Removal of a dorsal strut leads to a saddle deformity and removal of the anterior strut leads to tip collapse and columellar retraction.
  C F This may be essential in order to remove severe spurs.
  D T This is perfectly acceptable practice if the only problem is a crest displaced from the vertical position.
  E F Unilateral tearing of a torn mucoperichondrial flap is of little consequence and may, indeed, be beneficial in order to avoid a postoperative septal haematoma. However, efforts should be made to repair tears in both flaps if juxtaposed.

326 **Analgesia:**
- A   All non-steroidal anti-inflammatory drugs inhibit prostaglandin synthesis
- B   Aspirin prolongs the bleeding time
- C   Paracetamol overdose causes tinnitus
- D   Morphine causes diarrhoea
- E   Buprenorphine causes respiratory depression

327 **Grafts for head and neck reconstruction:**
- A   A random graft is a pedicled graft
- B   An axial graft is a pedicled graft
- C   A full-thickness skin graft is a pedicled graft
- D   Jejunum used to repair the pharynx is a pedicled graft
- E   The blood supply to an axial flap runs superficial to the underlying muscle layer

328 **The meninges:**
- A   The tentorium cerebelli lies between the two cerebellar hemispheres
- B   Cerebrospinal fluid flows beneath the pia mater
- C   The subdural space lies between the dura and the arachnoid mater
- D   Have no sensory innervation
- E   The pia mater is a vascular membrane

329 **Complications of suppurative otitis media:**
- A   All cases of sinus thrombosis are confined to the lateral sinus
- B   Papilloedema occurs following unilateral lateral sinus thrombosis
- C   Otitic hydrocephalus is usually associated with a sinus thrombosis
- D   A subdural abscess is an accumulation of pus between the dura mater and the skull
- E   The prime consideration of a subdural abscess is energetic treatment with high dose intravenous antibiotics

330 **Sarcoidosis:**
- A   May be diagnosed by an elevation in serum angiotensin converting enzyme levels
- B   Its lesions are caseating and granulomatous
- C   Usually produces an abnormal chest X-ray
- D   Tends to cause nasal obstruction when it affects the nose
- E   Produces red submucosal nodules in the nose

331 **Sinus osteomata:**
- A   Occur in 1% of routine sinus radiographs
- B   25% eventually became malignant
- C   Are commoner in Arabs
- D   May form part of the picture of Gardner's syndrome
- E   Are all ivory osteomata

326 A T They are all cyclo-oxygenase inhibitors.
     B T From both inhibition of thromboxane synthesis and impaired platelet aggregation and from reduced hepatic clotting factor synthesis.
     C F Although this effect is seen with aspirin overdose.
     D F Constipation occurs as a result of reduction in the motility of the gastrointestinal tract.
     E T It is reversed by naloxone only in very high doses.

327 A T It may be raised anywhere.
     B T An axial graft is based on a named arteriovenous pedicle.
     C F It is a free graft receiving its blood supply from the recipient site.
     D F It is a free graft, its blood supply being secured by microvascular anastomosis.
     E T A random flap has a poorer blood supply which it obtains from the subdermal plexus of its pedicle.

328 A F It covers the cerebellum and supports the cerebral occipital lobes.
     B F It circulates between the arachnoid and the pia mater.
     C T It is a potential space and contains a film of serous fluid.
     D F The dura mater is richly supplied with such fibres.
     E T It consists of a plexus of minute blood vessels held together by areolar tissue.

329 A F Most, but not all. There may be extension into the superior petrosal sinus or even into the cavernous sinus and jugular bulb.
     B F However, it will occur following a second and later contralateral sinus thrombosis and it is usually permanent.
     C T It occurs following the altered state of intracranial haemodynamics and is commoner in children and adolescents.
     D F The pus is situated between the dura and the arachnoid.
     E F Early surgical drainage is essential and is the prime consideration. However, intravenous antibiotic therapy may be instituted prior to surgery.

330 A T But levels must be very high and liver disease must be absent.
     B F Sarcoid is a non-caseating granulomatous disease.
     C T In 90% of subjects.
     D T
     E F Sarcoid involving the nose characteristically produces nasal obstruction and yellow submucosal nodules.

331 A T
     B F Malignant transformation is most uncommon.
     C T These people have a greater growth rate of the osteomata.
     D T Consisting of craniofacial osteomata, soft tissue tumours and colonic polyposis.
     E F They may be ivory or spongy.

332 **The blood supply of the nose is derived at least in part from:**
A Both the internal and external carotid arteries
B The ophthalmic artery
C The maxillary artery
D The facial artery
E The ascending pharyngeal artery

333 **ERA:**
A Stands for evoked response audiometry
B Brain stem evoked responses (BSER) can detect the auditory threshold
C Electrocochleography (ECochG) is a rapid and easily performed investigation
D Cortical electric response audiometry (CERA) is an invasive procedure
E To obtain postauricular myogenic responses requires sedation

334 **Immunoglobulin E:**
A Is detected in serum at concentrations of the order of 50 ng/ml
B Can fix complement
C Has a useful role in combating parasitic infections
D Has a molecular weight of 200 000
E Crosses the placental barrier

335 **Cricopharyngeal myotomy:**
A Should always be performed at the end of a horizontal partial laryngectomy
B Consists of division of the length of the inferior constrictor
C Should be performed as anteriorly as possible
D Is beneficial for dysphagia caused by neurological disease
E Should be performed routinely as part of excision of a pharyngeal pouch

336 **The eyeball:**
A Pupillary dilatation occurs via the sympathetic nervous system
B The anterior chamber contains aqueous humour
C The anterior and posterior chambers communicate with each other through the pupil
D The sclera is a thin well-vascularized membrane lining the posterior five-sixths of the eyeball
E The cornea is continuous with the sclera

337 **Non-organic hearing loss:**
A Can be diagnosed by cortical electric response audiometry
B Is diagnosed by the Stenger test
C The audiometrician may be at fault in the establishment of the diagnosis
D Does not occur in children
E The commonest presentation is a bilateral reduction in auditory threshold

332 A T The internal carotid artery supplies the anterior and superior portions
     B T via the anterior and posterior ethmoidal arteries. The external carotid
     C T system supplies the remainder via the maxillary artery, where the
     D T main nasal branches are the sphenopalatine and the descending
     E F palatine arteries.

333 A F It is more correctly known as electric response audiometry.
     B T But not as accurately as pure tone audiometry. They are more
            frequently used to detect lesions involving the auditory nervous
            system.
     C F It is a time-consuming hospital procedure involving numerous skilled
            workers and it is relatively costly.
     D F Values are obtained from surface electrodes on the vertex and ear.
     E F Measurements can be made in mobile, hyperactive or uncooper-
            ative children without the need for medication or a soundproof room.

334 A T And IgG at 12 mg/ml, IgM at 1 mg/ml and IgA at 2 mg/ml.
     B T Via its Fc portion.
     C T IgE levels are raised in the presence of parasitic infection and there
            is some evidence that atopics are relatively resistant to such infection.
     D T It has two light and two heavy chains.
     E F

335 A T Cricopharyngeal spasm postoperatively would predispose to
            aspiration.
     B F The thyropharyngeus is not divided.
     C F This would put the recurrent laryngeal nerves at risk.
     D T The suffering of many patients, so affected, may be eased.
     E T The development of a pharyngeal pouch is thought to be due to
            disordered cricopharyngeal function.

336 A T While constriction is made possible by the parasympathetic fibres
            carried in the oculomotor nerve.
     B T As does the posterior chamber.
     C T
     D F This describes the choroid. The sclera is the 'white' of the eye.
     E T Its laminae of fibrous tissue are transparent instead of white.

337 A T Although time-consuming, this method is very accurate.
     B T This test is based on the fact that with two identical sounds striking
            each normal ear there is an impression in one ear only if that one is
            nearer the sound.
     C T The patient may misunderstand the audiometric task, may be in-
            attentive or the meatus may be occluded by the audiometer earphone.
     D F But not as frequently as in adults.
     E F A unilateral deafness is more common.

338 **Nasal gliomas:**
    A   Maintain a connection with the subarachnoid space
    B   Are true neoplasms
    C   May be mistaken for an antrochoanal polyp
    D   Appear as red polypoidal masses that are firm and non-compressible
    E   The most common differential diagnosis is a dermoid cyst

339 **Indications for the osteoplastic frontal flap operation:**
    A   The removal of a large osteoma
    B   Chronically infected frontal sinus mucosa
    C   Exploration of the posterior wall of the frontal sinus after trauma
    D   Acute frontal sinusitis
    E   Removal of a recurrent mucocele

340 **Regulation of respiration:**
    A   Breathing stops if the spinal cord is transected above the origin of the phrenic nerves
    B   The respiratory centre for voluntary respiration is located in the pons and medulla
    C   Is independent of the vagus nerve
    D   The respiratory chemoreceptors are solely the aortic and carotid bodies
    E   Proprioceptors in muscles, tendons and joints stimulate the respiratory centre

341 **Causes of a fluctuating sensorineural hearing loss include:**
    A   Acoustic neuroma
    B   Suppurative labyrinthitis
    C   Menière's disease
    D   Meningitis
    E   Arachnoidal cysts

342 **The nasal cycle:**
    A   Occurs in 50% of subjects
    B   Has a frequency of 2–4 h
    C   Is modified by lying on one side
    D   Is the cause of alternating nasal obstruction seen in chronic rhinitis
    E   Causes a ten-fold variation of nasal resistance in an individual nasal cavity

338   A F Nasal gliomas are not continuous with the subarachnoid space or the central nervous system. If there is a connection, the lesion is an encephalocele. However, 15% of nasal gliomas do have a fibrous connection to the subarachnoid space.
       B F They are heterotopic brain tissue.
       C T
       D T
       E T

339   A T
       B T
       C T
       D F Acute frontal sinusitis is treated by intravenous antibiotics, maxillary sinus lavage and frontal sinus trephine.
       E T

340   A T The neurones innervating the respiratory musculature are totally dependent on the nervous impulses from the brain.
       B F This is the site of the involuntary (automatic) centre. The voluntary centre lies in the cerebral cortex.
       C F Afferents in the vagus nerves from lung receptors modify the output from the respiratory centre.
       D F There are also receptor cells in the medulla.
       E T This effect may help to increase ventilation during exercise.

341   A T This is an occasional finding in small tumours.
       B F The hearing loss is permanent.
       C T This is the most common and important disease of the inner ear causing a fluctuant sensorineural hearing loss.
       D F This hearing loss is irreversible.
       E T A rare cause.

342   A F The nasal cycle occurs in 80% of the population.
       B F The nasal cycle has a frequency of 30 min–4 h.
       C T Lying on one side causes ipsilateral nasal congestion and contra-lateral nasal decongestion. This is probably due to the hemihydrotic reflex where (sympathetic) sweating to the 'down' side is reduced while sweating to the 'up' side is increased. The nasal changes are a function of sympathetic tone.
       D T The effects of the nasal cycle are exaggerated when the nasal mucosa is congested.
       E T Total nasal resistance varies by a factor of two but the resistance of each nasal cavity varies by as much as ten-fold.

343 **Carcinoma of the larynx:**
  A   A subglottic tumour presenting with stridor should be treated by emergency laryngectomy
  B   A T_1 glottic neoplasm should be treated primarily with radiotherapy
  C   A glottic lesion with unilateral lymph nodes is more commonly treated with radiotherapy
  D   A horizontal partial supraglottic laryngectomy would be indicated for tumours of the epiglottis and/or vestibular folds
  E   A subglottic lesion with neither stridor nor involved palpable neck glands should receive radiotherapy initially

344 **The mucous membrane of the sinuses:**
  A   Is discontinuous with that of the nose and is termed mucoperiosteum
  B   Is basically ciliated pseudostratified columnar epithelium
  C   Contains very few goblet cells
  D   Is very thin
  E   Contains tracts of cilia interspersed with areas of few or absent cilia

345 **Surgery for otosclerosis:**
  A   Stapes mobilization is effective only in the short-term
  B   Nowadays, there is no place for a fenestration operation
  C   In a fenestration operation, fascia is placed over the created fistula in the lateral semicircular canal
  D   Otitis externa is a contraindication to stapedectomy
  E   The risk of total loss of hearing in the operated ear for a stapedectomy is 2%

346 **Rendu–Osler–Weber syndrome:**
  A   Has epistaxis as the most common symptom
  B   Always affects the nose to some extent
  C   Coagulation studies frequently demonstrate an abnormality
  D   The nasal lesions tend to lie directly beneath the nasal epithelium
  E   The most commonly occurring nasal lesion is a flat spider-like telangiectasis

347 **In rhinoplasty:**
  A   Periorbital ecchymoses occur as a result of performing lateral osteotomies
  B   Removal, reshaping and replacement of the nasal septum is accompanied by an unacceptably high rate of cartilage reabsorption
  C   When a dorsal nasal hump is removed, medial and lateral osteotomies should always be performed
  D   Medial osteotomies should curve somewhat laterally near the root of the nose
  E   The line of the lateral ostetomies in the nasomalar plane is usually obvious

343   A   T   If a tracheostomy is performed and it is not followed by an emergency laryngectomy then it is estimated that one in three patients will develop stomal disease.
      B   T   This dictum is generally accepted. Laser surgery is also accepted.
      C   F   Usual treatment is a total laryngectomy and a radical neck dissection, but radiotherapy for a T_1N_1 glottic lesion is a less common alternative.
      D   T   But not for tumours crossing the ventricle to involve the true vocal cords.
      E   T   Surgery should be reserved for residual or recurrent disease.

344   A   F   Sinus mucosa and nasal mucosa are in continuity.
      B   T
      C   F   Goblet cells are generally plentiful.
      D   T   The mucosa is very thin in the normal nose and is termed mucoperiosteum.
      E   T   There are tracts of ciliated cells which all beat towards the sinus ostia. Between these tracts, however, the mucosa is relatively poorly ciliated.

345   A   T   Re-ankylosis is a problem.
      B   F   It is of value in the presence of an abnormally situated facial nerve, a persistent stapedial artery or in cases of obliterative otosclerosis where reclosure has followed stapedectomy.
      C   F   A tympanomeatal flap is placed over the fenestra.
      D   T   Stapedectomy requires complete asepsis to be successful.
      E   T   The patient must be informed of this fact.

346   A   T
      B   F   The nose is not always affected and pure gastrointestinal forms do exist.
      C   F   Coagulation studies are normal since the disease is due to the absence of muscle and elastic tissue in the walls of the blood vessels.
      D   T   The weakness of the blood vessels gives rise to subepithelial lesions.
      E   T   Other types of lesion include pin-point purple spots and larger nodular telangiectases.

347   A   T   Following the elevation of the dorsal nasal skin, less severe ecchymoses also occur
      B   F   The nasal septum can be removed and replaced without fear of extrusion or necrosis.
      C   F   Only in most cases. In a narrow nose it would be better to use a cartilage graft to close the roof of the deformity caused by the removal of the hump. In a narrow nose, lateral osteotomies would tend to make the nose too narrow.
      D   T
      E   F   The line of the intended osteotomies in the nasomalar groove is often difficult to determine and, in many cases, requires considerable experience.

348 **Ossicular discontinuity:**
    A   Of traumatic origin most commonly affects the stapes
    B   When caused by chronic otitis media, the most frequent site of the discontinuity is at the long process of the incus
    C   An air–bone gap of up to 40 dB would be expected
    D   Measurement of the stapedial reflex is not possible in all cases
    E   Tympanometry exhibits a negative pressure within the middle ear space

349 **Mast cells:**
    A   Mast cell granules contain histamine as the major pharmacological mediator
    B   Mast cell granules contain prostaglandin D_2
    C   Liberate preformed and newly formed mediators on stimulation
    D   Mast cell degranulation is at least partly under neural control
    E   Require IgE to degranulate

350 **Behçet's disease:**
    A   Produces specific laboratory abnormalities
    B   Responds well to cyclophosphamide
    C   Presents with ulceration of the upper aerodigestive tract and of the genitalia
    D   Tends not to produce nasal septal ulcers
    E   Causes ocular inflammation and cutaneous vasculitis

351 **Complications of thyroidectomy:**
    A   Thyrotoxicosis
    B   Hypoglossal nerve injury
    C   Hypercalcaemia
    D   Hoarseness
    E   Hypothyroidism

352 **Lymphatic drainage of the head and neck:**
    A   The deep cervical lymph nodes are situated around the internal jugular vein
    B   All the lymph vessels of the head and neck drain into the deep cervical group of lymph nodes
    C   The tonsil drains to the jugulodigastric lymph node
    D   The tip of the tongue drains to the submental glands bilaterally
    E   The occipital region of the scalp drains to the postauricular lymph nodes

348   A F The most frequently affected ossicle is the incus.
      B T The blood supply is most precarious in the region of the long process, especially the lenticular process.
      C F It would be closer to 60 dB.
      D F It is possible when the discontinuity lies medial to the stapedius tendon, such as a fracture involving the stapedial crura. Such an isolated fracture, however, would be excessively rare.
      E F But the compliance value is raised.

349   A T Over half of the mast cell granule content is histamine.
      B F Prostaglandin D_2 is a newly formed mediator synthesized at the time of degranulation.
      C T These are released during mast cell degranulation.
      D T Mast cell degranulation is facilitated by α-receptor and cholinoceptor stimulation, and inhibited by β_2-receptor stimulation.
      E F Mast cells can degranulate in response to non-immunologic mechanisms, which include radiographic contrast media, venoms, morphine, dextran, and mechanical and thermal trauma.

350   A F No specific laboratory test is helpful.
      B F There is no adequate treatment although steroids may occasionally be useful.
      C T
      D F Nasal involvement consists of superficial septal ulcers, which may also occur in the postnasal space and range from 2 mm to 2 cm in size.
      E T

351   A T A 'thyroid crisis' is rarely seen nowadays. It occurs because of massive release of thyroxine from a hyperactive gland during surgery. Thyrotoxicosis may also develop in a thyroid remnant.
      B F The nerve does not lie within the surgical field.
      C F Although hypocalcaemia can occur following damage to or excision of the parathyroid glands.
      D T From damage to either recurrent laryngeal nerve.
      E T Usually due to excessive removal of thyroid tissue.

352   A T Lying from the base of the skull to the root of the neck.
      B T The efferents then form the jugular trunk.
      C T Situated below the posterior belly of digastric, between the angle of the mandible and the anterior border of sternomastoid.
      D T The remainder of the anterior two-thirds drains to the submandibular group of lymph nodes.
      E F Drainage is to the occipital nodes situated in the upper angle of the posterior triangle.

353 **Facial nerve grafting:**
  A   A cross-facial anastomosis involves anastomosing unimportant buccal and zygomatic branches on the healthy side to the mandibular and ocular branches on the paralysed side
  B   The sural nerve would be used for a cross-face anastomosis
  C   If insufficient nerve is available while attempting to join two ends in the region of the lateral semicircular canal, a graft must be taken
  D   A hypoglossal–facial anastomosis is useful where there is insufficient viable facial nerve proximal to the site of neural disruption
  E   The great auricular is the nerve most frequently used

354 **Anterior rhinomanometry:**
  A   Can be performed by nearly all patients
  B   Measures total nasal resistance directly
  C   Samples posterior nasal pressure by occluding and cannulating one nostril
  D   Requires a sampling tube to be placed along the nasal floor into the nasopharynx
  E   Can be performed by less patients than can posterior rhinomanometry

355 **Nasal plasmacytoma:**
  A   20% of extramedullary plasmacytomas occur in the head and neck
  B   Causes extensive bone destruction
  C   Produces nasal obstruction, rhinorrhoea and epistaxis
  D   Cervical lymph node involvement is common
  E   Responds reasonably well to radiotherapy

356 **Histology of the nasopharynx:**
  A   At 20 years of age the nasopharynx is lined almost solely by ciliated columnar epithelium
  B   After the age of 10 years 10% of the total mucosal surface is lined by squamous epithelium
  C   Transitional epithelium is usually found in some areas
  D   Melanocytes are rarely present
  E   Squamous metaplasia tends to occur only in smokers

357 **Otitis externa:**
  A   May be a localized manifestation of a generalized disorder
  B   An auroscopic diagnosis of infection with *Aspergillus niger* may be possible
  C   Furunculosis is invariably caused by a β-haemolytic streptococcus
  D   Can occur following intrameatal self-cleaning with cotton buds
  E   Otitis externa haemorrhagica spares the tympanic membrane

353 A T Nasolabial incisions are required to create a supralabial tunnel.
     B T Because, in this case, substantial length is required.
     C F Permanent anterior transposition of the nerve may allow an end to end anastomosis to be carried out.
     D T Unnecessary facial nerve fibres should be clipped in order to allow for preferential regeneration to the muscles of the eye and mouth. This principle should be applied to any extratemporal facial nerve graft.
     E T Because of its substantial length, accessibility and minimal effects resulting from its loss.

354 A T
     B F Airflow rate and pressure gradients are measured for each side of the nose in turn. The total nasal resistance is then calculated from the parallel resistance formula.
     C T
     D F The cannula pierces only the adhesive tape occluding the nostril and lies in the anterior naris.
     E F Anterior rhinomanometry can be performed by nearly all patients. Posterior rhinomanometry cannot be performed by approximately 30% of patients, making it useless for clinical work.

355 A F 80% of extramedullary plasmacytomas occur in the head and neck but nasal plasmacytomas are rare, accounting for less than 5% of the sinonasal tumours.
     B T
     C T
     D F Cervical lymph node metastases are uncommon.
     E T This should be considered as the first line of treatment.

356 A F At birth the nasopharynx is lined solely by ciliated columnar epithelium.
     B F By this time 60% of its total mucosal surface is lined by squamous epithelium.
     C T Occurring somewhere in between the two varieties of ciliated columnar and squamous epithelium.
     D F Melanocytes are found in all of the above types of epithelium.
     E F The cause of the squamous metaplasia is not known.

357 A T Such as psoriasis, seborrhoeic dermatitis or eczema.
     B T The black-headed conidiophores may be identified or there may be a black or grey membrane present.
     C F The usual pathogen is *Staphylococcus aureus*.
     D T The migratory desquamation process is interfered with and a cycle of events then occurs culminating in otitis externa.
     E F This condition is also known as acute bullous myringitis.

358 **Histoplasmosis:**
- A   Is caused by the fungus *Histoplasma capsulatum*
- B   Infection is caused by inhaling infected dust
- C   Tends to infect the nose as a primary site
- D   Causes pulmonary manifestations at an early stage
- E   Responds well to systemic penicillin

359 **Branchial cysts:**
- A   Usually have an internal opening
- B   The presenting symptom is usually intermittent swelling
- C   Usually protrude beneath the anterior border of the upper third of sternomastoid
- D   Are all cystic on palpation
- E   Treatment is invariably surgical

360 **In sphenoid sinus lavage:**
- A   The anterior wall of the sinus can usually be seen
- B   The correct point of puncture lies 5 cm from the anterior nasal spine
- C   The correct angle of approach is 60° from the line of the nasal floor
- D   The cannula should be positioned as near to the midline as possible
- E   The Watson–Williams blunt sphenoid trocar and cannula is used to cannulate the sinus ostium

361 **The palatine bone:**
- A   Includes the pterygoid plates
- B   Contributes to the formation of the orbit
- C   In the adult, the height of the perpendicular plate measures twice the transverse width of the horizontal plate
- D   The perpendicular plate forms part of the middle and inferior meatus of the nasal cavity
- E   The horizontal plate articulates with the alveolar process of the maxilla

362 **The infratemporal approach to the skull-base (Fisch):**
- A   Permanent anterior transposition of the facial nerve is carried out routinely
- B   Complete homolateral deafness is inevitable
- C   If there is intracranial tumour extension greater than 2 cm, a two-stage removal is preferred
- D   Employs blind sac closure of the external auditory canal
- E   Tumours of the anterior cranial fossa are accessible by this approach

358 A T
     B T Histoplasmosis is caused by inhaling soil dust infected with bat, bird or chicken faeces.
     C F
     D T The disease tends to affect the lungs first. Upper airway manifestations include ulcers on the tongue, buccal mucosa and larynx.
     E F The treatment of choice is amphotericin B.

359 A F Only the minority have such an opening although, in theory, this should always be present.
     B F The swelling is continually present in 80% of patients.
     C T
     D F Only 70% are cystic; 30% feel solid.
     E T A search should be made for a tract and an internal opening.

360 A F It is most unusual to see the anterior wall of the sinus.
     B F
     C F The correct point of puncture lies 7 cm from the anterior nasal spine at an angle of 45° from the line of the nasal floor.
     D F The cannula should be positioned in the same vertical plane as the posterior end of the middle turbinate since the sinus wall is thinner at this point. It tends to be quite thick in the midline.
     E F It is used to puncture the anterior wall of the sinus and not to cannulate the ostium, which is usually small and may be multiple.

361 A F These form part of the sphenoid bone.
     B T Its orbital process helps to constitute the floor.
     C T At birth they are about equal.
     D T
     E F It articulates with the palatine process of the maxilla.

362 A T A groove is cut from the anterior epitympanum across the root of the zygoma.
     B F Only a permanent conductive deafness results due to obliteration of the middle ear cleft.
     C T This reduces the mortality rate.
     D T Which helps to avoid the damage of postoperative infection and allows for primary healing of the wound.
     E F Areas that are accessible by this approach include the jugular foramen, the petrous apex, the clivus, and the parasellar and parasphenoid compartments.

363   **Pollen counts:**
  A   Are expressed as number of grains per m^3 of air
  B   Are higher in moist damp weather
  C   Are made by depositing pollen grains on a glass slide using various methods and counting the grains with a microscope
  D   Can be used in conjunction with weather forecasts to give a pollen count forecast
  E   Pollen count forecasts have been found to be useful in the management of hay fever

364   **Choanal atresia:**
  A   Has an incidence of 1 in 20 000 live births
  B   Occurs twice as often on the right side as on the left
  C   Is commoner in males
  D   Other congenital abnormalities occur in 10% of unilateral cases
  E   Other congenital abnormalities occur in 20% of bilateral cases

365   **Of nose and sinus tumours:**
  A   55% occur in the maxillary antrum
  B   10% occur in the nasal cavity
  C   10% occur in the ethmoids
  D   5% occur in the frontal sinus
  E   5% occur in the sphenoid sinus

366   **The epiglottis:**
  A   Is composed of hyaline cartilage
  B   Has an attachment to the hyoid bone
  C   Is essential for deglutition
  D   The vallecula is the depression on either side of the median glosso-epiglottic fold
  E   The aryepiglottic fold contains muscle fibres

367   **Otitis media:**
  A   Cholesteatoma can occur in the presence of chronic suppurative otitis media
  B   Cholesteatoma can occur in the presence of chronic non-suppurative otitis media
  C   Tuberculous otitis media is usually secondary to pulmonary tuberculosis
  D   In acute non-suppurative otitis media the effusion is usually mucoid
  E   Acute suppurative otitis media is an infection of the mucoperiosteal lining of the middle ear cleft by pyogenic organisms

368   **Nasal resistance to airflow:**
  A   Decreases with exercise
  B   Decreases with anxiety
  C   Increases following alcohol ingestion
  D   Increases when water enters the nose
  E   Increases with high humidity

363 A T
    B F They are higher in warm dry windy weather.
    C T This is but one of several ways of making the count.
    D T If the pollen count for the day is correlated with the weather forecast, a pollen count forecast can be made for the next day.
    E F Pollen count forecasts tend to be inaccurate (like weather forecasts)!

364 A F It occurs in 1 in 5000 live births.
    B T When the disease is unilateral.
    C F It is commoner in females.
    D F
    E F Other congenital abnormalities occur in 45% of unilateral cases and in 60% of bilateral cases.

365 A T Most studies of nose and sinus cancer report the following figures:
    B F 55% maxillary sinus, 35% nasal cavity, 9% ethmoids and 1% from
    C T the remaining sinuses.
    D F
    E F

366 A F It is composed of yellow elastic fibrocartilage.
    B T The hyo-epiglottic ligament is attached to the upper border of the hyoid and its lateral extension raises a ridge of mucous membrane, the pharyngo-epiglottic fold (lateral glosso-epiglottic fold), bilaterally.
    C F Normal deglutition can take place in the absence of the epiglottis.
    D T Situated between the tongue anteriorly and the epiglottis posteriorly.
    E T Of the same name, which form part of the sphincter of the laryngeal inlet.

367 A T This is usual.
    B T Unresolved middle ear effusion is thought to be a predisposing factor in the development of a cholesteatoma.
    C T Infected cough particles ascend the eustachian tube.
    D F It is more likely to be serous, thin and runny. The thicker secretion occurs more commonly in chronic non-suppurative otitis media.
    E T This is its definition.

368 A T Exercise produces a linear decrease in nasal resistance up to 120 W for 5 min. This is a function of sympathetic tone.
    B T Anxiety reduces nasal resistance because of a rise in sympathetic tone and circulating catecholamines. The nose is 5 times more sensitive than the heart to the latter agents.
    C T Alcohol is a generalized vasodilator – and this includes the nose. It causes an increase in nasal resistance.
    D T Water entering the nose may produce the diving reflex seen in all mammals. This includes an increase in nasal resistance and also forced expiration, glottic closure, an increase in lower airway resistance, bradycardia, various changes in blood pressure and vasoconstriction in all organs except the brain and heart.
    E F Humidity has no effect on nasal resistance.

369 **Reinke's oedema:**
  A   Can affect any region of the larynx
  B   Is always bilateral
  C   Is also known as dysphonia plicae ventricularis
  D   Is best treated by voice rest
  E   Consists of an accumulation of fluid in the loose subepithelial space of the vocal cords

370 **Lymphatic drainage of the nasopharynx:**
  A   The lymphatic tissue of Waldeyer's ring drains into the upper deep cervical lymph nodes
  B   The lymphatic tissue of Waldeyer's ring drains into the lymph nodes of the retrostyloid compartment of the parapharyngeal space
  C   The nasopharynx has a rich submucosal lymphatic plexus
  D   The nasopharyngeal submucosal lymphatic plexus drains into medial and lateral retropharyngeal lymph nodes
  E   The upper deep cervical lymph nodes drain to the posterior triangle

371 **The cochlear nerve:**
  A   Enters the brain stem at the upper border of the pons
  B   Proximal to the cochlear nucleus most of its nerve fibres cross the midline
  C   Carries some motor fibres
  D   Its terminal fibres end in contact with the hair cells
  E   Most of the afferent neurones end at the inner hair cells

372 **Aspirin sensitivity is associated with:**
  A   Nasal polyposis
  B   An elevated serum anti-aspirin IgE
  C   Asthma
  D   Intolerance to tartrazine
  E   Non-eosinophilic non-allergic rhinitis

373 **Relapsing polychondritis:**
  A   Affects the cartilage of the ears, nose, larynx, trachea, ribs, joints and eustachian tubes
  B   Is not associated with a sensorineural hearing loss
  C   Causes florid changes in the nasal mucosa
  D   Can be diagnosed by the identification of a specific anti-cartilage antibody
  E   Causes inflammation of the cartilage of the nasal dorsum, eventually resulting in a saddle nose deformity

374 **Adenocarcinoma of the nose and sinuses:**
  A   Accounts for up to 20% of nose and sinus malignant tumours
  B   Usually starts in the ethmoid sinuses
  C   Tends to extend into the maxillary sinus
  D   Carries a worse prognosis than squamous cell carcinoma
  E   Is relatively slow-growing

369   A   F   It is limited to the glottis.
      B   F   Usually, but not always.
      C   F   In the latter, phonation occurs using the false vocal cords.
      D   F   Treatment is surgical and uses microlaryngeal techniques, often with the aid of the carbon dioxide laser.
      E   T   This is Reinke's space.

370   A   T   The lymphatic drainage of the nasopharynx is complex and is divided
      B   T   into two: (1) Waldeyer's ring (adenoids, tubal tonsil, lymphoid tissue
      C   T   in the fossa of Rosenmüller, islands of lymphatic tissue in the naso-
      D   T   pharynx, palatine and lingual tonsils) which drains into the lymph
      E   F   nodes in the retrostyloid compartment of the parapharyngeal space and then to the upper deep cervical nodes; and (2) a submucosal lymphatic plexus draining to the retropharyngeal lymph nodes, then to the posterior triangle and upper cervical nodes.

371   A   F   The cochlear nerve enters the brain stem at the upper border of the medulla, close to the inferior cerebellar peduncle.
      B   T   They ascend in the lateral lemniscus.
      C   F   Although the nerve carries both afferent and efferent nerve fibres, it is not a motor nerve.
      D   T
      E   T   Only a minority, which cross the tunnel of Corti in its lower part, are associated with the outer hair cells.

372   A   T   8% of such patients exhibit aspirin intolerance.
      B   F   Aspirin sensitivity is not an allergic phenomenon.
      C   T   The triad of aspirin intolerance, nasal polyposis and asthma is well known.
      D   T   Patients with aspirin intolerance cross-react to several other chemicals, including the azo dyes. Of the latter, tartrazine is the one most commonly seen.
      E   F   Aspirin sensitivity is associated with eosinophilic vasomotor rhinitis rather than the non-eosinophilic variety.

373   A   T
      B   F   It is also associated with episcleritis and anaemia.
      C   F   The disease has little or no effect on the nasal mucosa.
      D   F   Although it is probably an autoimmune disease, no anti-cartilage antibody has been detected.
      E   T

374   A   F   Adenocarcinomas account for about 8% of nose and sinus malignant neoplasms.
      B   T
      C   T
      D   F   The 3-year survival rates are: adenocarcinoma 50%, squamous cell carcinoma 20%.
      E   T

375 **Muscles attached to the mandible include:**
  A   Buccinator
  B   Depressor labii inferioris
  C   Mentalis
  D   The superior constrictor
  E   Stylohyoid

376 **Radiology of the ear:**
  A   A Stenver's view demonstrates the whole length of the petrous bone
  B   A lateral oblique view of the mastoid differentiates between the internal and external auditory meatus
  C   A Towne's view looks only at one ear
  D   A submentovertical view demonstrates the middle ear well
  E   The facial canal is well demonstrated by conventional radiography

377 **Chronic bacterial sinusitis may be associated with the following organisms:**
  A   Anaerobes can be cultured in nearly all cases
  B   *Veillonella* species
  C   *Peptococcus* species
  D   *Corynebacterium acnes*
  E   5% of cases are due to aerobic organisms

378 **Radical neck dissection:**
  A   Involves clearance of the lymphatic area between the midline and the anterior border of trapezius
  B   Involves clearance of the lymphatic area between the level of the hyoid and the clavicle
  C   Levator scapulae can be rotated anteriorly to protect the carotid tree
  D   Levator scapulae should be sutured superiorly, if rotated, to the posterior belly of digastric
  E   If rotated, levator scapulae should be sutured inferiorly to the periosteum over the clavicle

379 **The external nose:**
  A   The contribution of the nasal bones to the nasal pyramid is relatively constant
  B   The upper lateral cartilages almost always underlie the alar cartilages
  C   The nasion is the midline point where the nasal bones meet the frontal bones
  D   The rhinion is the midline point where the nasal bones meet the upper lateral cartilages
  E   The nasal spine of the frontal bone overlies the nasal bones

375 A T Along the anterior border of the ramus.
    B T Below the mental foramen.
    C T Just above the mental protuberance.
    D T Above the mylohyoid ridge.
    E F

376 A T
    B F They are superimposed.
    C F A comparison of both petrous apices is possible.
    D T It gives the best plain X-ray assessment of its air content, degree of translucence and the ossicular chain.
    E F The Stenver's view, which may show the descending part, is probably the only projection of value. CT scanning is far superior.

377 A T Chronic sinusitis is basically a disease dominated by anaerobic organisms.
    B T
    C T
    D T These are all important anaerobes implicated in chronic sinusitis.
    E F About 30–40% of cases are probably associated with mixed aerobic infection.

378 A T
    B F The area for clearance extends from the skull-base and mandible superiorly to the clavicle inferiorly.
    C T Especially in the irradiated patient.
    D T
    E F Inferiorly it is sutured to the stump of the sternomastoid.

379 A F The contribution of the nasal bones to the external nasal pyramid is very variable.
    B F The upper lateral cartilages underlie the alar cartilages in 70% of cases but in 30% of cases they either overlie or approximate end to end with the alae.
    C T
    D T The nasal bones are attached to each other by a midline suture. Where this suture meets the frontal bone is termed the nasion. Where this suture meets the upper lateral cartilages is termed the rhinion.
    E F The nasal bones are supported in their attachment to the frontal bone by the underlying nasal spine of the frontal bone.

380 **Cerumen:**
- A   Is solely the product of the ceruminous glands
- B   Contains a high concentration of lipid
- C   The average human ear contains between 1000 and 2000 ceruminous glands
- D   Ceruminous glands are present throughout the external auditory canal
- E   Ceruminous glands are sparse in Orientals

381 **Nasal mucociliary transport is decreased by:**
- A   Cystic fibrosis
- B   Smoking
- C   Viral infections
- D   Adenoidectomy
- E   Cocaine

382 **Ameloblastoma:**
- A   Occurs 5 times more commonly in the mandible than in the maxilla
- B   Histologically bears a resemblance to the enamel organ of the tooth
- C   Occasionally metastasises
- D   May be confused with adenoid cystic carcinoma
- E   Requires a wide surgical excision

383 **The optic nerve:**
- A   Has no Schwann cells
- B   The optic chiasma is attached to the anterior part of the floor of the third ventricle
- C   All of its fibres decussate at the optic chiasma
- D   A lesion of one optic tract immediately proximal to the optic chiasma is likely to cause a homonymous hemianopia
- E   In the orbit is supplied by the ophthalmic artery

384 **The mastoid:**
- A   The anterior end of the digastric ridge indicates the position of the stylomastoid foramen
- B   The area where the bony covering of the sigmoid sinus flattens while passing medially is known as MacEwen's triangle
- C   The sigmoid sinus passes deep to the facial nerve
- D   The mastoid process is present at birth
- E   Most people have a cellular type of mastoid

385 **The following can be used to assess nasal patency:**
- A   Anterior and posterior rhinomanometry
- B   Whole body plethysmography
- C   The Glatzel plate
- D   The Zwaardemaker mirror
- E   Nasal peak inspiratory flow

380   A F It is a mixture of the secretory products of the ceruminous and sebaceous glands.
      B T Mostly contributed by the sebaceous glands.
      C T
      D F They are not present in the inner bony portion.
      E T The wax is of the 'dry' type in Orientals. The 'wet' type is found in Caucasians and Negroes.

381   A T The visco-elastic properties of the mucous blanket are deranged.
      B T
      C T Virus infections cause loss of cilia.
      D F Adenoidectomy has been shown to improve mucociliary transport where the adenoid tissue was diseased.
      E T Cocaine causes temporary ciliary damage.

382   A T
      B T
      C F The tumour is locally malignant and behaves a bit like a basal cell carcinoma. It does not metastasize.
      D T
      E T There tends to be reabsorption of bone at the growing edge and thus the tumour may be larger than radiological examination would suggest.

383   A T It is identical with the white matter of the central nervous system and has no power of regeneration when divided.
      B T
      C F Only the nasal fibres of each side do this.
      D T While a lesion centred on the chiasma, such as a pituitary adenoma, would be likely to cause a bitemporal hemianopia.
      E T And distally by the central artery on its way to the retina.

384   A T This landmark may be used to locate the facial nerve during mastoid surgery.
      B F This area is known as Trautmann's triangle.
      C T Prior to entering the jugular bulb below the hypotympanum.
      D F Thus the facial nerve leaving the skull is relatively superficial.
      E T Approximately 80%.

385   A T Both of these measure nasal resistance to airflow.
      B T This method, which is used to measure pulmonary resistance, is performed with the mouth open and the nose occluded, and then with the mouth closed while breathing through the nose. The difference is equal to the nasal resistance.
      C T
      D T Both of these rely on the condensation of exhaled water vapour onto a cold surface. It is useful clinically to judge nasal airflow but gives little objective indication of nasal resistance to airflow.
      E T Peak nasal airflow gives a moderately good assessment of objective nasal patency. Although not very accurate, it is probably useful in the clinical environment since it is very quick and easy to perform.

386 **Labyrinthitis:**
- A   Prompt treatment of suppurative labyrinthitis will usually result in at least some recovery of auditory function
- B   In suppurative labyrinthitis the associated vertigo is usually not severe
- C   In paralabyrinthitis the bony covering of the membranous labyrinth becomes thinned which then becomes progressively sensitive to caloric stimuli
- D   Nystagmus occurs when a fistula sign is thought to be weakly positive
- E   Serous labyrinthitis is a retrospective diagnosis

387 **Lupus vulgaris:**
- A   Does not involve the nasal mucous membrane
- B   Causes considerable scarring
- C   *Mycobacterium tuberculosis* is easily cultured from biopsy material
- D   Caseating granulomata on histological examination are diagnostic
- E   Produces brown raised nodular lesions on the skin

388 **Olfaction:**
- A   All olfactory cells respond to all odours to some extent
- B   The stimulation of an olfactory receptor cell is associated with calcium ion influx into the cell
- C   All odorant molecules must interact with mucus overlying the receptor cells for coding and transduction to occur
- D   The odours of foods show preference shifts throughout the day
- E   Children less than 4 years of age are aware of aesthetic differences in odours

389 **Recognized surgical treatments for Menière's disease include:**
- A   Transtemporal (middle fossa) approach for vestibular nerve section
- B   Cochlear nerve section
- C   Grommet insertion
- D   Fenestration of the lateral semicircular canal
- E   Surgery should be reserved for severely disabling disease

390 **Surgery for laryngeal paralysis:**
- A   Teflon injection is useful in the presence of stridor
- B   Teflon injection is used in the presence of a bilateral vocal cord paralysis with a weak voice
- C   Teflon should be injected into the margin of the true vocal cord
- D   Arytenoidectomy is useful for improving the voice in bilateral vocal cord paralysis
- E   Arytenoidectomy is always performed by an external approach

386   A   F Once pus formation has occurred there will be complete and irreversible loss of vestibular and cochlear function.

       B   F It is extremely severe and incapacitating.

       C   T A 'fistula' into the lateral semicircular canal is not an uncommon discovery during mastoid surgery.

       D   F Nystagmus occurs when the sign is strongly positive. In a weakly positive test the patient complains of vertigo but nystagmus is absent.

       E   T In serous labyrinthitis there is hyperaemia but not pus formation. The distinction between serous and suppurative labyrinthitis depends on whether there is recovery of vestibulocochlear function and this can only be assessed retrospectively.

387   A   F Lupus vulgaris involving the external nasal skin commonly extends to the nasal vestibule and may involve the nasal mucosa.

       B   T Scarring is more severe than in tuberculosis.

       C   F The organism is very difficult to demonstrate in this disease.

       D   F Caseation is unusual.

       E   T

388   A   F Although the mechanism of olfactory coding is not completely understood, it is thought probable that different groups of olfactory cells respond to different odours and that no cell responds to all odours.

       B   T

       C   T Otherwise olfactory coding is not possible.

       D   T The judgement of food odorant pleasantness varies with satiety but the intensity of the odour is not affected.

       E   F Such children do not express a preference as regards pleasantness and unpleasantness to different odours, although they have no difficulty perceiving each odour.

389   A   T This would allow for the preservation of any remaining hearing.

       B   T This may relieve the tinnitus.

       C   T There appears to be some symptomatic relief.

       D   F This is of no proven value.

       E   T As no surgical option can guarantee success.

390   A   F The stridor would then worsen.

       B   F It is performed for unilateral paralysis, enabling the functioning vocal cord to reach across and phonate against the paralysed vocal cord.

       C   F At least 2.5 mm lateral to the cord margin.

       D   F Arytenoidectomy separates the vocal cords and would be useful for unilateral cord paralysis in adduction and in midline fixation. Quality of voice is worsened in exchange for an improvement in the airway.

       E   F Although external surgery is the commoner method by the frontal and lateral approaches, endoscopic removal is also possible.

391 **Nasal mucosal mast cells:**
- A Are a different type of cell to those found in connective tissue
- B Are inhibited from degranulating by disodium cromoglycate
- C Orchestrate the early events seen in allergic rhinitis
- D Are stimulated to divide by interleukin-2
- E Bind IgE by its Fc portion

392 **Squamous carcinoma of the sinuses:**
- A Ethmoidal tumours usually present with ophthalmic symptoms
- B Has a better prognosis when occurring in the frontal sinus
- C Radiotherapy is probably best given prior to radical surgery
- D Causes frank epistaxes
- E Antral tumours present most commonly with oral symptoms

393 **In rhinoplasty:**
- A The nasal tip is considered to be formed as a system of geodesic triangles
- B The nasal tip is supported by the nasal septum
- C The supratip region is partly supported by the nasal septum
- D A more natural shape to the nose is achieved by allowing the nasal bones to lie underneath the frontonasal processes
- E Lateral osteotomies carried out with a 2 mm osteotome via separate lateral stab incisions are associated with less risk of a 'floating' nasal bone than when carried out using a saw

394 **The cerebellum:**
- A The two cerebellar hemispheres are joined by the lingula
- B The inferior cerebellar peduncle connects the cerebellum to the pons
- C The superior cerebellar peduncle connects the cerebellum to the pons
- D Purkinje cells are found throughout the central nervous system
- E Is related anteriorly to the medulla, pons and third ventricle

395 **Causes of cochlear hydrops include:**
- A Menière's disease
- B Syphilis
- C Paget's disease
- D Multiple sclerosis
- E Benign positional vertigo

391 A T There are two types of mast cell – the mucosal and the connective
        tissue types. They differ both morphologically and histochemically.
        Mucosal mast cells are unaffected by sodium cromoglycate.
     B F Disodium cromoglycate only inhibits connective tissue mast cells
        from degranulating.
     C T The mast cell is central to the allergic response, responding to
        immune stimulation and producing the mediators of inflammation.
     D F Interleukin-1 is sensitized by macrophages and activates helper T
        cells. Interleukin-2 is sensitized by helper T cells and activates further
        T cells and killer T cells. Interleukin-3 is produced by macrophages and
        causes mast cells to divide.
     E T The Fc portion of IgE binds to specific IgE Fc receptors on the mast
        cell membrane.

392 A F The incidence of presenting symptoms for ethmoidal neoplasms is:
        55% nasal, 32% ophthalmic, 5% facial and 8% other.
     B F Such tumours of the frontal and sphenoidal sinuses carry a worse
        prognosis.
     C T
     D F This is unusual and a sanguinous rhinorrhoea is more common.
     E F The incidence of presenting symptoms for antral neoplasms is:
        39% facial, 34% nasal, 14% oral, 9.5% ophthalmic and 3.5% other.

393 A T A system of flat triangles formed together to make a dome.
     B F
     C T Although, theoretically, the cartilaginous external nose is self-
        supporting without the septum, in practice too much removal of the
        septum is followed by supratip depression.
     D T Achieved by performing a medial osteotomy curving somewhat
        laterally near the root of the nose.
     E T Lateral osteotomies carried out with the saw and curved chisel tend
        to separate the nasal bones from the periosteum, allowing the bones
        to float. The nasal bones may then fall into the pyriform aperture.
        When lateral stab incisions are used the periosteum is spared and the
        nasal bones remain attached, allowing the bone to hinge medially on
        the periosteum at the site of the lateral osteotomy.

394 A F They are joined by the vermis.
     B F It connects to the medulla.
     C F It connects to the back of the midbrain.
     D F Throughout all vertebrates these highly differentiated cells are found
        only in the cerebellar cortex.
     E F The fourth ventricle lies anteriorly.

395 A T There is generalized distension of the membranous labyrinth.
     B T Affecting the cochlear duct, the saccule and the utricle.
     C F
     D F
     E F

396 **Kartagener's syndrome:**
- A   Accounts for 10% of subjects suffering from primary ciliary dyskinesia
- B   Is associated with situs inversus
- C   Is associated with dextrocardia
- D   Is associated with chronic sinusitis
- E   Is not associated with secretory otitis media

397 **Chronic non-specific laryngitis:**
- A   Hyperplastic chronic laryngitis is associated with an increased likelihood to develop malignancy
- B   Pachydermia most commonly affects the junction of the anterior third and posterior two thirds of the glottic aperture
- C   May develop from unresolved acute laryngitis
- D   Is associated with chronic sinusitis
- E   Is commoner in males

398 **Terminal nasal trigeminal efferents conduct:**
- A   All the nasal parasympathetic nerve fibres
- B   All the nasal sympathetic nerve fibres
- C   Motor fibres to levator labii alaeque nasi
- D   Motor fibres concerned with dilating the nares in inspiration
- E   Fibres to the organ of Jacobsen in some mammals

399 **Investigation of vestibular function:**
- A   Frenzel's spectacles improve visual acuity
- B   Nystagmus provoked by positional testing may not be significant
- C   Unterberger's test gives better localization than does the Romberg test
- D   Optokinetic nystagmus is a normal phenomenon
- E   The Dundas–Grant caloric test utilizes water at body temperature

400 **Wegener's granulomatosis:**
- A   Is a systemic disease
- B   Tends to present as a persisting upper respiratory tract infection
- C   Involves the lung, kidney and skin
- D   Is associated with a raised ESR, anaemia and raised serum creatinine
- E   Is a type of lymphoma

396   A   F   Primary ciliary dyskinesia is associated with Kartagener's syndrome in 50% of cases.
     B   T   Correct functioning of cilia is necessary for rotation of the gut. If no cilia are functioning there is a 50% chance of the gut rotating either way.
     C   T
     D   T   Primary ciliary dyskinesia leads to male infertility, bronchiectasis, sinusitis and chronic bacterial rhinitis.
     E   F   Glue ear is a further association.

397   A   T   The occurrence of malignancy is higher in smokers.
     B   F   It mainly affects either the area of the vocal process of the arytenoid or the interarytenoid area.
     C   T   But it is more commonly a disorder of insidious onset.
     D   T   Chronic sinusitis can cause continual laryngeal irritation as a result of a postnasal drip.
     E   T   Like most laryngeal disease.

398   A   T   The parasympathetic nerve fibres run in the nasal divisions of the trigeminal nerve.
     B   F   Sympathetic nerve fibres accompany the blood vessels.
     C   F   This muscle is innervated by the facial nerve.
     D   F   The nostrils are dilated by facial muscles supplied by the facial nerve.
     E   F   The organ of Jacobsen is said to be innervated by the nervi terminales (the so-called XIII cranial nerve). These nerves run with the olfactory nerves and then course down the nasal septum to the organ of Jacobsen. It is not present in human beings.

399   A   F   There is practically no visibility as they consist of 15–20 dioptre lenses. However, they do reduce optic fixation.
     B   F   It is always an abnormal finding.
     C   T   The number of degrees of deviation can be measured over a period of time.
     D   T   It may be observed by watching a passenger's eyes in a moving train looking out of a window at telegraph poles.
     E   F   Cooled air is pumped into the external auditory meatus. This method of caloric testing is useful in the presence of a tympanic membrane perforation.

400   A   T   It is basically a vasculitis.
     B   T   It tends to present as a slowly resolving upper respiratory tract infection. By about the second month, however, the nasal symptoms include an increasing serosanguinous nasal discharge followed by foul-smelling blood-stained crusts. Vague nasal pain is common and nasal examination shows friable nasal mucosa.
     C   T
     D   T
     E   F

401 **Eosinophils:**
- A   Are recruited by eosinophilic chemotactic factor of anaphylaxis (ECF-A) secreted by mast cells
- B   Help to moderate the early response of immediate hypersensitivity
- C   Help to produce the late phase of immediate hypersensitivity
- D   Their presence in nasal secretions is diagnostic of allergic rhinitis
- E   Are present in large numbers in nasal polyps

402 **Chordomas:**
- A   60% occur in the region of the skull-base
- B   May present with nasal obstruction, a feeling of nasal fullness and deafness
- C   Arise from vestigial notochordal remnants
- D   Cause extensive bone destruction
- E   Complete excision is often impossible

403 **The laryngeal skeleton:**
- A   The cricoid is a complete cartilaginous ring
- B   The inferior cornua of the thyroid cartilage lie free
- C   The arytenoid cartilages lie on the lateral part of the superior border of the arch of the cricoid
- D   The anterior border of the thyroid lamina is fused with that of the opposite lamina at an angle of 120° in men
- E   The cuneiform cartilages lie anteriorly to the corniculate cartilages

404 **Primary objectives of surgical treatment for chronic suppurative otitis media:**
- A   Restoration of hearing
- B   Maintenance of the posterior meatal bony wall
- C   Promotion of middle ear ventilation
- D   Prevention of complications
- E   Treatment of complications

405 **Normal nasal flora include:**
- A   Corynebacteria
- B   Staphylococci
- C α-haemolytic streptococci
- D β-haemolytic streptococci
- E   *Aspergillus*

406 **Osteoradionecrosis:**
- A   Will usually occur if a partial mandibulectomy is performed in a patient who has previously received radiotherapy to this area
- B   Radiotherapy causes dental caries
- C   Necessary dental extractions should be performed in the first week following radiotherapy
- D   Is caused by an effect on the blood supply of the bone
- E   Does not affect the maxilla

401   A T ECF-A is a preformed mediator liberated by mast cells during degranulation.
      B T Eosinophils secrete histaminase (which inhibits histamine), aryl-sulphatase (which inactivates leucotriene $C_4D_4E_4$) and phospholipase D (which inactivates platelet activating factor).
      C T Eosinophils secrete eosinophil cationic protein which helps in the late phase response.
      D F Eosinophils are present not only in allergic rhinitis but also in the eosinophilic type of vasomotor rhinitis.
      E T Nasal polyposis occurs in eosinophilic vasomotor rhinitis in 30% of such patients. Nearly all patients with nasal polyposis have eosinophilic vasomotor rhinitis.

402   A F Chordomas can occur anywhere along the spine but one third occur in the skull-base region. These present in the nasopharynx.
      B T
      C T
      D T
      E T

403   A T It is the only complete cartilaginous ring throughout the entire air passages.
      B F They articulate with the cricoid at a synovial joint.
      C F They are so-placed but are on the lamina of the cricoid.
      D F The angle of fusion is 90° in men and 120° in women.
      E T The former lying in the aryepiglottic folds and the latter articulating with the apex of each arytenoid.

404   A F This is of secondary importance.
      B F Not at the expense of safety.
      C F This is also of secondary importance.
      D T By removing polypi, granulations, diseased bone and cholesteatoma, and allowing aeration and drainage of mastoid air cells.
      E T Whether they be intracranial or intratemporal, as well as making the ear safe. Other aims include the prevention of further deterioration of function and cessation of discharge.

405   A T
      B T Some 20–50% of subjects are carriers of *Staphylococcus aureus*.
      C T
      D F
      E F

406   A T
      B F But it does predispose to periodontal disease which in turn causes caries.
      C F They should be performed before commencing radiotherapy.
      D T The blood supply is altered making the bone more prone to infection.
      E F It affects the maxilla but neither as often nor as severely as it affects the mandible.

407 **Systemic nasal decongestants:**
    A   Are useful in short courses at controlling obstructive symptoms in acute infective rhinosinusitis
    B   Are not associated with tachyphylaxis
    C   Do not cause rhinitis medicamentosa
    D   Do not reduce nasal resistance to airflow in chronic rhinitis
    E   Are beta-adrenoceptor agonists

408 **Physiology of hearing:**
    A   The axis of rotation of the malleus and incus is in a line parallel to the malleus handle and incus long process
    B   The stapedius muscle contracts in response to sound pressure levels 50 dB or greater above threshold
    C   The tympanic membrane vibrates in a manner similar to a simple stretched elastic membrane
    D   Endolymph in the scala media has a positive potential relative to that of perilymph
    E   Cochlear microphonics represent changes in endocochlear potential

409 **Howarth's operation:**
    A   As originally described employs a near horizontal infra-orbital skin incision
    B   Is advocated in acute ethmoiditis without complications
    C   Is advocated in cases of chronic ethmoidal sinusitis
    D   Is advocated in cases of recurrent nasal polyposis
    E   Is probably safer than intranasal ethmoidectomy

410 **Polymorphic reticulosis:**
    A   Is clinically similar to Wegener's granulomatosis
    B   May develop into a lymphoma
    C   Is a systemic disease
    D   Tends not to cause nasal ulceration
    E   Is treated with cyclophosphamide and steroids

411 **The acquired immunodeficiency syndrome (AIDS):**
    A   Kaposi's sarcoma does not affect the face
    B   Malignant lymphoma is the second commonest malignant tumour affecting patients with AIDS
    C   Presentation with a lung disorder accounts for approximately 25% of cases
    D   *Pneumocystis carinii* accounts for 85% of pulmonary infections
    E   The drug of choice for *Pneumocystis carinii* infection is erythromycin

407 A T Systemic nasal decongestants reduce nasal resistance by causing nasal mucosal vasoconstriction.
     B F Tachyphylaxis occurs if the agents are used for long periods.
     C T
     D F
     E F Systemic nasal decongestants, like topical decongestants, are α-receptor agonists.

408 A F It is approximately parallel to a line drawn as a tangent to the upper edge of the pars flaccida.
     B F It responds to sound 80 dB or greater above threshold.
     C F Each portion of the tympanic membrane has its own degree of displacement, occurring maximally near the lower margin.
     D T The endocochlear potential is $+80$ mV.
     E F Summating potentials represent such changes. Cochlear microphonics originate in the hair cells and accurately follow the pattern of the sound stimulus.

409 A F There are two similar operations for the approach to the frontal and ethmoidal sinuses. Howarth's operation utilizes a near-vertical paranasal skin incision and Patterson's operation uses a near-horizontal infra-orbital incision. In practice, most surgeons use a combination of the two.
     B F It is advocated in acute ethmoiditis with complications which have not resolved with systemic antibiotic therapy.
     C T
     D T
     E T Especially in inexperienced hands. The intranasal approach, although safe in experienced hands, is difficult to master and has few landmarks.

410 A T Polymorphic reticulosis is the disease most often confused with Wegener's granulomatosis.
     B T Histologically, there is a dense infiltrate of immature and angiocentric lymphoid cells. The disease may, in fact, be a localized lymphoma or may progress to become a lymphoma.
     C F The disease only affects the nose in contrast to Wegener's granulomatosis which affects other organs.
     D F It is locally destructive and initially causes nasal ulceration.
     E F The treatment is with radiotherapy.

411 A F It may affect practically any area of the skin as well as internal organs.
     B T Second only to Kaposi's sarcoma.
     C F Such infection accounts for over 50% of all initial presentations.
     D T Patients usually have a 6–8 week history of dyspnoea and dry cough often associated with a fever.
     E F It is co-trimoxazole.

412 **Sinonasal tumours:**
- A   Myxomas are of ectodermal origin
- B   Control of angiosarcoma is difficult
- C   Haemangiopericytomas are found relatively frequently in the head and neck
- D   Local recurrence of haemangiomas does not usually occur after removal
- E   Capillary haemangiomas tend to occur on the lateral nasal wall

413 **The soft palate:**
- A   Separates the oropharynx from the nasopharynx
- B   Is covered throughout by stratified squamous epithelium
- C   Contains taste buds
- D   Palatopharyngeus elevates the larynx and pharynx
- E   The uvula has no glands

414 **Pure tone audiometry:**
- A   For air-conducted sound thresholds the symbol X is used for the left ear
- B   For bone-conducted sound thresholds the symbol [is used for the left ear
- C   For air-conduction threshold testing the first sound used should be 250 Hz
- D   The threshold of hearing for a particular frequency is that intensity which cannot be heard following the previous positive response
- E   The better hearing ear is usually tested first

415 **Topical nasal steroids:**
- A   If used at recommended doses produce slight adrenal suppression over a long period
- B   Do not cause nasal candidiasis
- C   May cause epistaxis
- D   Are not as potent at producing a fall in nasal resistance as antihistamines in allergic rhinitis
- E   Are effective at controlling nasal polyposis in cystic fibrosis

416 **Excision of the superior portion of the alar cartilages will:**
- A   Tend to narrow the nasal tip
- B   Tend to elevate the nasal tip
- C   Tend to cause tip collapse
- D   Tend to lead to alar collapse during inspiration
- E   Tend to cause nasal obstruction by making the limen nasi more pronounced

417 **Granulomatous disorders which affect the larynx include:**
- A   Blastomycosis
- B   Leprosy
- C   Amyloid
- D   Diphtheria
- E   Non-healing (Stewart's) granuloma

154 Answers

412 A F Myxomas are of mesenchymal origin and are rare in the head and neck. When they do occur, however, the maxillary antrum is the commonest site.
  B T This is reflected in the poor 10-year survival of 15%.
  C T Accounting for 25% of their total.
  D F The lesion should be widely excised with a cuff of muco-perichondrium, otherwise recurrence will occur.
  E F The capillary haemangioma produces the 'bleeding polyp of the septum'.

413 A T
  B F Its upper border is covered with respiratory epithelium.
  C T On its inferior surface.
  D T Thus helping to shorten the pharynx during swallowing.
  E F The uvula is a mass of mucous glandular tissue.

414 A T O is used for the right ear.
  B F It is used for the right ear and] is used for the left ear.
  C F It should be 1000 Hz since this is easily identified as sound.
  D F It is the lowest intensity heard on 50% of occasions on repeated crossings (down 10 dB, up 5 dB, etc.).
  E T

415 A F Topical nasal steroids do not cause adrenal suppression in recommended doses.
  B T Although oral candidiasis is associated with topical steroids taken to treat asthma.
  C T Epistaxis is not an uncommon side-effect. However, its occurrence demands cessation of the steroid spray.
  D F Topical nasal steroids reduce nasal resistance more effectively than do antihistamines.
  E F The polyps of cystic fibrosis contain neutrophils, not eosinophils. They are, therefore, probably different from classical ethmoidal polypi.

416 A T
  B T
  C F
  D F
  E F

417 A T Laryngeal blastomycosis is usually secondary to the pulmonary disease.
  B T
  C F This is not a granulomatous disorder.
  D F Occasionally, diphtheria is found in the larynx, but again, this is not a granulomatous disorder.
  E F This is not known to affect the larynx.

418   **The nasal septum:**
    A   Most authorities believe that the nasal septum is formed from at least four bones
    B   The vomerine/maxillary crest articulation is long in early life
    C   The caudal nasal septal cartilage does not extend beyond the nasal spine
    D   The septal cartilage/ethmoid articulation is 'end to end'
    E   The septal cartilage/maxillary crest articulation is 'tongue and groove'

419   **Facial nerve disorders:**
    A   Hemifacial spasm is invariably bilateral
    B   Melkersson's syndrome consists of a facial nerve palsy associated with a swollen parotid gland
    C   Facial paralysis occurs in Sjögren's syndrome
    D   A facial paralysis may complicate infectious mononucleosis
    E   Electroneuronography requires at least one fully functional facial nerve for the result to be meaningful

420   **Perennial rhinitis:**
    A   Causes symptoms in 10–15% of the population
    B   Is usually controlled by topical nasal steroids
    C   Only occasionally requires surgical treatment
    D   Is not associated with radiological changes in the paranasal sinuses
    E   Is rarely associated with bronchial hyper-reactivity

421   **The parasympathetic supply to the nose:**
    A   Arises from the superior salivatory nucleus
    B   Runs in the lesser superficial petrosal nerve
    C   Reaches the nose via the Vidian nerve
    D   Relays in the sphenopalatine ganglion
    E   May be interrupted in an operation to relieve rhinorrhoea

422   **The external auditory canal:**
    A   In the adult is approximately 2.5 cm in length
    B   Runs a straight course
    C   The outer two thirds is cartilaginous
    D   The junction of the bony and cartilaginous sections forms the narrowest part of the canal
    E   The sensory nerve supply to the posterior half is from the vagus nerve

418 A T The nasal septum is made up from the quadrilateral cartilage, the vomer, the perpendicular plate of the ethmoid, the palatine bone and the maxillary crest.
 B F Early in life this articulation is cartilaginous and only gradually ossifies.
 C F The caudal septal cartilage projects beyond the nasal spine within the columella.
 D T
 E T

419 A F As its name implies, it invariably affects the muscles on one side of the face only.
 B F Its features are recurring attacks of facial palsy, lip swelling and congenital furrowing of the tongue.
 C F There is no known association.
 D T Or mumps.
 E T Since the number of degenerated fibres is expressed as a percentage compared to the normal side.

420 A T However, only 2–4% require regular treatment.
 B T
 C T A few may require reduction of the turbinates.
 D F Eosinophilic vasomotor rhinitis is frequently associated with sinus infection and mucosal thickening is frequently seen in allergic and perennial rhinitis.
 E F Bronchial hyper-reactivity is almost always associated with perennial rhinitis even in the absence of chest symptoms.

421 A T
 B F
 C T
 D T It is then conducted via the greater superficial nerve, which joins the deep petrosal nerve to form the Vidian nerve, which then supplies the nose after relay in the sphenopalatine ganglion.
 E T Vidian nerve neurectomy is carried out by dividing or coagulating the Vidian nerve in the pterygopalatine fossa. It is useful in reducing severe rhinorrhoea in non-eosinophilic vasomotor rhinitis that has been unresponsive to other therapy.

422 A T From the bottom of the concha to the tympanic membrane.
 B F It runs a tortuous S-shaped course which helps serve as protection to the tympanic membrane.
 C F It is cartilaginous in its outer third and bony for its inner two thirds.
 D F The isthmus is the narrowest point, situated midway along the bony portion, 5 mm from the tympanic membrane.
 E T Via its auricular nerve (of Arnold).

423 **Nasal dermoid cysts:**
A   Contain skin appendages
B   Their creation is an embryonic fault between the developing nasal bones and the cartilaginous capsule
C   May be superficial small lesions
D   May occur with an associated dermal sinus
E   Any associated dermal sinus is a superficial lesion

424 **The nasal mucosal sinusoids:**
A   Fill and empty causing mucosal swelling and shrinkage, resulting in changes in nasal resistance to airflow
B   The venous sinusoids vasoconstrict when adrenaline is applied to the nose by a direct action on contracting circular vascular smooth muscle
C   The degree of venous sinusoid filling is controlled by cushion veins
D   The cushion veins have an adrenergic innervation only
E   Produce a histological picture similar to a cavernous haemangioma

425 **Pharyngeal repair:**
A   A gastric pull up requires two anastomoses
B   A colonic transplant requires two anastomoses
C   A radial forearm flap is based on the radial artery
D   A deltopectoral flap includes muscle
E   A free jejunal segment is useful for tumours that extend into the thoracic oesophagus

426 **Temporal bone fractures:**
A   80% are longitudinal
B   Most CSF leaks require surgical closure
C   Are not always evident on radiological examination
D   Antibiotics should be administered in the presence of CSF otorrhoea
E   May produce vertigo

427 **Ipratropium bromide:**
A   Is a cholinoceptor agonist
B   Is an alpha-adrenoceptor antagonist
C   Is useful at controlling the symptoms of severe rhinorrhoea in non-eosinophilic non-allergic rhinitis
D   Is administered topically as a spray
E   Is effective at controlling the symptoms of allergic rhinitis

423   A   T But epidermal inclusion cysts, sometimes included in this category, only contain epidermal elements.
      B   T
      C   T
      D   T
      E   F Dermoid cysts can occur with or without a sinus. Those occurring with a sinus are extensive and deep-seated while those without a sinus tend to be superficial.

424   A   T It is the degree of distension or filling of the sinusoids that governs the degree of nasal mucosal swelling and thus nasal resistance.
      B   F The sinusoids themselves contain little or no muscle and are thus unresponsive to adrenaline.
      C   T So-called cushion veins are located at the distal end of the venous sinusoid. They have a very thick longitudinal muscular wall. When this contracts in response to a reduction in sympathetic outflow or an increase in parasympathetic outflow, the vein 'bunches' up and occludes its lumen, allowing the proximal venous sinusoid to distend. With the converse stimulation the cushion vein relaxes, its lumen opens, the sinusoid empties and the nasal mucosa decongests.
      D   F
      E   T

425   A   F An anastomosis is required at the pharyngeal end only.
      B   F Three are required – a pharyngeal, a gastric and a colonocolonic.
      C   T Preoperative testing of the suitability of the ulnar artery to supply the whole hand is required.
      D   F It is a pedicled skin flap only.
      E   F Stomach or colon would then be chosen.

426   A   T 20% are transverse.
      B   F Most will spontaneously cease within 7–10 days.
      C   T The diagnosis is frequently a clinical one.
      D   T To reduce the possibility of meningitis.
      E   T It is usually transient but may persist as benign positional vertigo.

427   A   F
      B   F It is a cholinoceptor antagonist, as is atropine.
      C   T It is very useful in perennial non-allergic rhinitis that is unresponsive to steroids.
      D   T The recommended dose is two sniffs in each nostril four times each day (20 μg/sniff).
      E   F It has little or no effect in allergic rhinitis.

428 **The sympathetic nerve supply to the nose:**
    A   Is regulated by the hypothalamus
    B   Relays in the superior cervical (stellate) ganglion
    C   Reaches the nose by two routes
    D   Partly runs in the deep petrosal nerve
    E   Relays in the sphenopalatine ganglion

429 **Congenital deformities of the nasal septum:**
    A   Occur less frequently with non-elective caesarean section than with spontaneous vaginal delivery
    B   Only 20% of adults have a straight nasal septum
    C   Damage to the nasal septum occurs at birth rather than *in utero*
    D   May cause feeding problems and cyanotic attacks
    E   May take the form of a widened nasal septum

430 **Subglottic stenosis:**
    A   The predominant symptom is stridor
    B   Is increasing in incidence
    C   Congenital subglottic stenosis is usually diagnosed at birth
    D   An Evans laryngotracheoplasty is the operation of choice for acquired subglottic stenosis
    E   Most affected children will require definitive surgery

428 A T

    B T

    C F The sympathetic supply to the nose probably arises from the hypothalamus and is transmitted via the thoracolumbar spinal cord to the superior cervical sympathetic ganglion where it relays. From here, the sympathetic nerves enter the nose by at least four routes – the nasolacrimal nerve, the maxillary nerve, the Vidian nerve and with blood vessels.

    D T

    E F It relays in the superior cervical ganglion. The parasympathetic fibres relay in the sphenopalatine ganglion.

429 A F Spontaneous vaginal delivery and non-elective caesarean section produce the same rate of deviated nasal septa, whereas elective caesarean section tends to protect the nose.

    B T

    C F Damage to the septum can occur at birth and *in utero*. The acute effects in the neonatal period of congenital nasal septal deviations have probably been overstated. However, a large proportion of patients presenting with a deviated nasal septum have probably had the problem since birth. Nasal septum deformities tend to lead gradually to mucosal hypertrophy and this accounts for the late presentation of most patients.

    D T A severe deviated nasal septum in a neonate can give rise to feeding problems and cyanotic attacks.

    E T Bimalar pressure on the head of the baby tends to force the palate upwards and compress the nasal septum leading to an S- or C-shaped septal deformity. If the pressure is severe enough, the septum may be widened.

430 A T Above all others, including failure to thrive.

    B T The acquired type is increasing in incidence as more premature babies survive who require intubation.

    C F Only in severe cases. It more commonly presents several months later following a respiratory tract infection.

    D F A laryngotracheal reconstruction, using a free graft of costal cartilage, is required because acquired subglottic stenosis is frequently associated with cricoid perichondritis.

    E F Only the minority require definitive surgery. A tracheostomy may be all the surgical treatment that is required and the symptoms may decrease as the child grows.

431 **The following are allergies (mast cell degranulation mediated by IgE):**
  A   Sensitivity to cotton dust (byssinosis)
  B   Hypersensitivity to morphine
  C   Hypersensitivity to radiological contrast media
  D   Aspirin intolerance
  E   Hypersensitivity to nickel (contact dermatitis)

432 **Vestibular neuronitis:**
  A   Is caused by a virus
  B   Occurs mostly between 30 and 50 years of age
  C   Includes cochlear symptoms
  D   The lesion is thought to lie between the labyrinth and the
        vestibular nuclei
  E   Recovery is usually complete

431   A F
      B F
      C F Mast cells not only degranulate in response to immunological stimuli but also in response to other stimuli including: physical trauma and temperature change, pharmacological agents (such as radiological contrast media, morphine and dextran) and cotton dust.
      D T Aspirin intolerance is not an immunological phenomenon. Aspirin inhibits cyclo-oxygenase and, in some patients, the reduction in prostaglandin synthesis may allow the effects of leucotrienes to occur unopposed. Their effects include bronchoconstriction, oedema and chemotaxis.
      E T Nickel is a hapten and combines with normal body protein, the combination being allergenic.

432   A F The aetiology is obscure.
      B T The sexes are involved equally.
     ·C F Symptoms are purely vestibular.
      D T As there is neither auditory nor central nervous system involvement.
      E T In most people there is full recovery within 1 month. Treatment is purely symptomatic.